MA Review

Exam Certification
Pocket Guide

THIRD EDITION

MA Review

Exam Certification
Pocket Guide

THIRD EDITION

Susan M. Perreira, MS, RMA

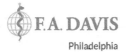

F.A. DAVIS

Philadelphia

F. A. Davis Company

1915 Arch Street
Philadelphia, PA 19103
www.fadavis.com

Printed in the United States of America

Last digit indicates print number: 10 9 8 7 6 5 4 3 2

Senior Publisher: T. Quincy McDonald
Content Project Manager: Julie Chase
Director of Content Development: George W. Lang
Art and Design Manager: Carolyn O'Brien

Library of Congress Control Number
2021945625

To my husband Dave
for his understanding, encouragement,
and support through this process.

To all of my students
who entrusted me with their education
in this wonderfully diversified field
and inspired me to create this book.

Preface

Joy! That is the best word to describe the feeling I have each time a medical assisting graduate lets me know that my pocket guide and online review were both essential to achieving their national certification. Having been certified as a medical assistant through the American Association of Medical Assistants (AAMA) and the American Medical Technologists (AMT), I know the feeling of accomplishment that credentialing gives someone. This book has been my opportunity to prepare medical assistants for that all-important credential they have been striving to earn. Because of objectives established by the Centers for Medicare & Medicaid Services (CMS) in promoting interoperability (PI), it is now more important than ever to become credentialed in the medical assisting field.

Because so many of you have let me know that my book played an important part in preparing you for your credentialing examination, I've now created a third edition to help new students and MAs who want a quick review source. It covers all of the MA examination's required comprehension areas: law and ethics, laboratory procedures, clinical skills, pharmacology, medical terminology, anatomy and physiology, common diseases, oral and written communication, emergencies, front office procedures (scheduling, reception, human relations, insurance, coding), office management (payroll, accounting, bookkeeping), and much more.

This study guide retains its concise outline format to provide essential information without all the fluff. It is small enough to easily travel with, so you can refer to it whenever you have time throughout the day. You can use the provided spaces to add study notes to personalize it.

Here is what's new:

- Chapters are now grouped according to the three main areas of study: General, Administrative, and Clinical knowledge.

- Chapter 1 provides information about preparing for the following exams:
  - Certified Medical Assistant [CMA (AAMA)]
  - Registered Medical Assistant (RMA)
  - Certified Medical Administrative Specialist (CMAS)
  - National Certified Medical Assistant (NCMA)
  - National Certified Medical Office Assistant (NCMOA)
  - Medical Administrative Assistant Certified (MAAC)
  - Medical Assistant Certified (MAC)
  - Clinical Medical Assistant Certified (CMAC)
- Each chapter begins with an introduction highlighting the relevancy of the topic in the exams.
- New illustrations are included throughout the book.
- Study tips are given, beginning in the first review chapter (Law & Ethics) for use throughout your study.
- Each chapter ends with 3 review questions. For more, access Davis Edge.
- All information, such as changes in pharmacology, technology, communication, and recent diseases/conditions, has been updated to match changes in the medical field.

Davis Edge Online Test Bank

MA Review provides Davis Edge online quizzing with review questions to give you an opportunity to test your knowledge. More test questions have been added, and all questions include rationales for correct answers. In addition, the online quizzing provides candidates wishing to test themselves in specific subject areas (terminology, ICD coding, phlebotomy, medical records, scheduling, etc.) the ability to do so.

Additionally, the online test bank also allows one to create 5-, 10-, or 20-question quizzes that can be filtered by exam type, including CMA, RMA, CMAS, NCMA, NCMOA, MAAC, MAC, and CMAC. These quizzes can be scored, with correct answers and rationales given when errors have been made. You may retest at any time.

As a former MA faculty member and experienced administrative and clinical MA, I recognize the knowledge that newly graduated and experienced MAs must possess to become properly credentialed and, later, recredentialed. Most medical assisting graduates have passed their certification exam on their first try, and I hope that, with the help of this *MA Review*, third edition, you will pass the examination your first time, too.

Good luck!

Brief Contents

Contents

Part Two: ADMINISTRATIVE

Part 1

General

Chapter 1

Medical Assistant Certification

Are you currently employed as a medical assistant (MA)? Are you about to graduate or have recently graduated from a medical assisting education program?

If you are employed, it is very important that you become credentialed right away if you want to stay employed. If you are graduating, credentials will help you be a good candidate for your new career as an MA. Today's medical employers recognize the value of credentialed MAs and seek them out for the following reasons:

- The physician's electronic health record (EHR)/electronic medical record (EMR) system requires that only the credentialed MA can enter patient information. It's the law.
- Employee professionalism is essential.
- Credentialed MAs present a lower liability risk in several areas of their practices.
- The practice of medicine is increasingly complex.
- Credentialed MAs make valuable ongoing contributions to the clinical and administrative sides of a given practice through continued education and recertification.

Being a credentialed MA is fast becoming a requirement for employment because of the ever-increasing restrictions brought about by the Health Information Technology for Economic and Clinical Health Act (HITECH). Under this law, hospitals, doctors, and health-care professionals can qualify for Medicare and Medicaid incentive funds when they adopt and meaningfully use certified EHR technology.

The term *"meaningful use"* referred to a set of EHR/EMR performance criteria broken out across several stages. In 2019 the need to expand on *"meaningful use"* led to a new name: Promoting Interoperability (PI). This now included the health data exchange among providers, such as public health and clinical data exchange, e-prescribing, provider-to-patient exchange, and health information exchange. Each stage has core objectives, and measures for those objectives have been established by the Centers for Medicare & Medicaid Services (CMS).

The CMS imposed an important condition; the MA must be credentialed from an organization other than the MA's employer. This represents a significant achievement for credentialed MAs. The CMS has recognized the particularly significant role played by certified MAs in the healthcare delivery system and the qualities that set them apart from other allied health personnel.

To obtain the MA credential, you must successfully pass an examination administered by a nationally accredited agency, either the National Commission for Certifying Agencies (NCCA) or the American National Standards Institute (ANSI), not your employer. The American Medical Technologists (AMT) association, the American Association of Medical Assistants (AAMA), the American Medical Certification Association (AMCA), and the National Center for Competency Testing (NCCT) are accredited by the NCCA.

The Benefits of Credentialing

- Employers are looking for credentialed MAs!
- Attainment of this credential confirms your in-depth knowledge of medical assisting and demonstrates your dedication to this field.
- The yearly income for a certified MA (Certified Medical Assistant [CMA], Registered Medical Assistant [RMA], Certified Medical Assistant Specialist [CMAS], National Certified Medical Assistant [NCMA], National Certified

Medical Office Assistant [NCMOA]), Medical Administrative Assistant Certified (MAAC), Medical Assistant Certified (MAC), or Clinical Medical Assistant (CMAC) is higher than the employee wages of uncertified MAs.

- Networking with other certified MAs, while earning continuing education units (CEUs), may be cultivated by attending national conventions, state conventions, and local chapter meetings.
- With national certification, there is no need to apply for reciprocity if you move out of state and wish to continue working in the field.

Preparing for the Examinations

Study Tips

The more prepared you are for the examination, the more confident you will be. Getting started on the path to study is usually much more difficult than the actual studying itself. Once you've started down the path, you're on your way to earning that coveted credential!

- Create your own place to study, preferably quiet, with few or no interruptions, at a time when you are functioning well. It should be comfortable—but not too comfortable.
- Set up a study schedule for yourself and stick to it. **Commit, commit, commit!** Use 1.5 to 2 hours per day for consecutive days for a particular subject area (office, laboratory, clinical, anatomy, pharmacology, etc.).
  - Avoid cramming; it just puts too much pressure on you.
  - Organize your study time for each subject area.
  - Review competency skills.
- Take notes (especially on information you have forgotten).
- Create an outline format for your note taking. Outlining helps to organize your thoughts.
- Take notes in your own words to help you practice memorization.
- Highlight the key terms that will trigger your memory of the topic.

- Repetition helps memorization. You may want to use a digital recorder as an additional way to help you. Reciting the material you recall and then hearing the information you recorded incorporate audio learning into your studying.
- Once you have studied an area (pharmacology, law and ethics, etc.), review the area again to help reinforce your learning. **Be overprepared!**
- When you believe you know material in a chapter, **test yourself on that chapter!**
- A reminder to you has been inserted at the end of each chapter or major section.

Examination-Taking Tips

- Just remember…you know this information; you learned it in school and may be using a great deal of it already in your externship or medical assisting employment.
- Drive and time the trip to the testing center a few days in advance to remove any anxiety about the center's location and the time it will take to get there. Plan to arrive early the day of the examination; you'll avoid being late because of traffic jams, etc.
- The night before the examination, gather all the items you will need to bring with you to the examination (required identification[s], erasers, pencils, hard candy, etc.).
- The credentialing examinations are presented in a multiple-choice format, and you must choose an answer among 4 or 5 lettered response options. The AMT gives you 4 response options for the RMA and CMAS examinations. The AAMA gives you 5 response options. The NCCT gives you 4 response options for the NCMA and NCMOA examinations. The AMCA gives you 4 response options for the MAAC, MAC, and CMAC examinations.
  - Read each question and remember not to make assumptions by reading into the information presented. In other words, base your answer on the information provided.
  - Answer the question in your head before looking at the given response options.

- Read the question a second time for full comprehension and then view the response options.
- Remember, your initial response is usually the correct one unless you did not fully comprehend the question.
- If 2 or 3 response options are correct, check to see whether the last given option is an "all the above" or a combination of previous options.
- Incorrect response options are called distractors. Usually, after ruling out the obviously incorrect options, you will be left with 2 possible answers; select the most correct answer.
- Pay special attention to questions containing words that have been **bolded,** *italicized,* underlined, or CAPITALIZED.
- Watch out for words such as *except, unless, unacceptable, avoid, contraindicated,* or *never* that are used in a test question. These questions have a negative orientation; look for the single "negative" or "false" answer. The following is an example of this type of question:

The 5 Cs of communication components are all the following except:

A. consistent
B. clear
C. cohesive
D. concise
E. complete

   In this case you need to identify which responses are components of communication to find the one response that is not. The response that is not a component is the correct answer.

- You will encounter questions throughout the certification examinations that require critical thinking. This means that you will be problem-solving using logic to select the best solution to the situation in the question.
  - For example, you know the definition of *"triage,"* but you may be asked to apply triage to a given scenario posed to you in the multiple-choice question.

- The following is an example of a critical thinking question:

You are employed at an OB/GYN practice. The physician has confirmed a suspected pregnancy of one of your spouse's relatives. The relative nervously lets you know that no one in your spouse's family knows about this office visit. The most appropriate response is:

A. "If someone asks, I'll only tell them you had an office appointment."
B. "Be assured in knowing that I don't discuss or share any patient information outside of the office."
C. "Trust me, I'll only tell my spouse."
D. "This is such happy news; it should be shared."
E. "You should be very happy about this."

This question presents a situation in which you must decide the best way to respond. It is testing your ability to recognize your professional responsibility in ensuring that a patient's needs are appropriately met.

- Remember that this is a timed examination, so you need to spend less than a minute on each question. If the question asked lacks clarity for you, skip it. If you have enough time remaining at the end of the examination, go back to it.
- Be sure to answer ALL the questions; any question left unanswered will be scored as a wrong response.
- Last, but certainly not least, remember to relax! You've been studying hard and you know the answers. If you feel yourself tensing up during your examination, here's a little technique that works. Lick your lips and inhale quietly and slowly through your mouth. Concentrate on that cool sensation—it's relaxing. Now get back to the examination with a more relaxed and open mind. You may want to practice this relaxation technique while you are using the Edge product to create simulated examinations. You know the answers; use your knowledge and logical thinking!

The Examination Application Process

American Medical Technologists (AMT)

1. Applications may be downloaded from the AMT website (www.americanmedtech.org), completed, and submitted with required documentation and a certified check.
2. The AMT processes the application and then notifies the applicant to select a computer testing center from an approved list. Pearson Professional Centers are the testing sites for the RMA and CMAS certifying examinations.
3. The applicant contacts the center to arrange a convenient test date and time. MA education institutions also may serve as computer testing centers on AMT approval.
4. For application questions, www.americanmedtech.org or call (847)823-5169.

American Association of Medical Assistants (AAMA)

1. Applications must be completed and submitted with required documentation and a certified check.
2. The AAMA processes the application and then sends a scheduling permit to the applicant.
3. The applicant must contact an approved Prometric Test Center (www.prometric.com) to schedule the examination within 30 days of receipt.
4. The applicant will be limited to 3 attempts to obtain the credential.
5. For application questions, e-mail certification@aama-ntl.org or call 1-800-228-2262 or 1-312-899-1500.

National Center for Competency Testing (NCCT)

1. You may register on the NCCT website to complete the test application and receive processing examination approval online for a faster turnaround time.

2. Paper applications may be downloaded from the NCCT website (www.ncctinc.com), completed, and then submitted with required documentation and a certified check, money order, or charge card information.
3. The NCCT processes the application within a few days and then notifies the applicant.
4. The applicant chooses a test date by contacting an NCCT-approved test site. The testing centers are colleges and business schools that offer computerized examinations and testing on paper.
5. Applicants are allowed a maximum of 3 lifetime attempts for any single certification.
6. For application questions, visit www.ncctinc.com or call 1-800-875-4404.

American Medical Certification Association (AMCA)

1. If you have an account, log in and go to: Exam Registration.
2. If you do not have an AMCA account, go online to www.amcaexams.com/student-registration and set up an AMCA profile.
3. Complete the online registration form. You can use a charge card to secure your exam date and time.
4. Candidates are allowed 3 attempts to successfully pass the exam within the first year of the first exam, after which they can reapply 1 year from the date of their initial exam attempt.
5. For application questions, visit www.amca.com or call 1-888-960-2622.

AMT National Examinations to Earn RMA/CMAS Credentials

- Examinations are timed.
- Each examination consists of 210 multiple-choice questions with 4 choices for each question (A through D).

- Each question is weighted in value (1/4 point to 1 full point).
- A minimum score of 70 is required to pass.
- Applicants will know immediately on completion of the computerized examination whether they have earned the RMA/CMAS credential.

Content Outline of RMA Examination

Knowledge Area	Approx. % of Exam	Topics
General	41%	Anatomy and physiology, medical terminology, medical law and ethics, human relations, patient education
Administration	24%	Insurance, financial and bookkeeping, medical receptionist/secretarial/clerical
Clinical	35%	Asepsis, sterilization, instruments, vital signs and mensurations, physical examinations, clinical pharmacology, minor surgery, therapeutic modalities, laboratory procedures, electrocardiograms, first aid

Source: American Medical Technologists. AMT Candidate Handbook: Registered Medical Assistant (RMA). http://www.americanmedtech.org/files/RMA%20Handbook.pdf.

Content Outline of CMAS Examination

Knowledge Area	Approx. % of Exam	Topics
Medical assisting foundations	13%	Medical terminology, anatomy and physiology, law and ethics, professionalism

Continued

Knowledge Area	Approx. % of Exam	Topics
Basic clinical	8%	Patient history, charting, vital signs, asepsis
Clerical	10%	Scheduling, patient communication, patient information, community resources
Records management	14%	Systems, procedures, confidentiality
Insurance processing, billing, coding	17%	Same as Knowledge Area
Financial management	17%	Bookkeeping and office accounting, banking, payroll
Information processing	7%	Computing and its applications
Office management	14%	Communications, business organization, human resources, safety, supplies and equipment, physical site, risk management, quality assurance

Source: American Medical Technologists. Certified Medical Administrative Specialist (CMAS) Candidate Handbook. http://www.americanmedtech.org/GetCertified.aspx#177229-prepare-for-exam.

AAMA National Examination to Earn CMA Credential

- The examination is timed.
- The examination consists of 200 questions with 5 choices for each question (A through E); 20 of the 200 are "pre-testing questions" (preselected, not scored).
- The applicant will receive an immediate unofficial pass/fail result and will formally know whether he or she has

earned the CMA credential approximately 12 weeks after
completing the examination.

Content Outline of CMA Examination

Knowledge Area	Approx. % of Exam	Topics
General	36%	Medical terminology, anatomy and physiology, psychology, professionalism, communication, medicolegal guidelines and requirements
Administrative	28%	Data entry, office equipment, computer concepts, records management, screening and processing mail, scheduling and monitoring appointments, resource information and community services, office environment, policies and procedures, practice finances, accounting and banking
Clinical	36%	Infection control, treatment area, patient preparation and assisting physician, patient history interview, collecting and processing specimens, diagnostic testing, preparing and administering medications, emergencies, first aid, nutrition

Source: American Association of Medical Assistants CMA (AAMA). Certification/Recertification Examination Content Outline. aama-ntl.org.

NCCT National Examinations to Earn NCMA/NCMOA Credentials

- The examinations are timed.
- The NCMA examination consists of 150 multiple-choice questions with 4 choices for each question (A through D).

- The NCMOA examination consists of 186 multiple-choice questions with 4 choices for each question (A through D).
  - Each question and/or section is weighted in value.
  - A minimum score of 70 is required to pass.
- Applicants will know immediately on completion of the computerized examination whether they have earned the NCMA/NCMOA credential. If they are completing the examination on paper, results will be given in 4 to 6 weeks.

Content Outline of NCMA Examination

Knowledge Area	Approx. % of Exam	Topics
Anatomy and physiology	10%–12.5%	Body systems and functions; basic disease recognition; bones; body positioning for examination; major muscles
Medical office management	18%–20.5%	General office procedures, 10%–12.5%; bookkeeping, 4%; insurance processing, 4%
Infection and exposure control	12.5%	Biohazardous waste disposal; exposure control; asepsis; personal protective equipment; universal precautions; sanitation, sterilization, disinfection; OSHA safety regulations
Patient examination	10%–12.5%	Patient history and screening; basic examination skills; minor surgical assisting; wound care; therapeutic modalities assisting, vision and specialty testing; normal and abnormal condition recognition; patient instruction; first aid and cardiopulmonary resuscitation; scope of practice recognition

Knowledge Area	Approx. % of Exam	Topics
Phlebotomy	10%–12.5%	Venipuncture and capillary puncture; patient and site preparation; safety and infection control; equipment and tubes; coagulation and anticoagulation
Diagnostic testing	10%–12.5%	CLIA-waived laboratory testing; quality control and instrument maintenance; specimen collection; electrocardiographic testing, monitoring, and troubleshooting; basic respiratory testing, treatment
Medical terminology	10%–12.5%	Foundation of word structure; standard medical/pharmaceutical abbreviations and symbols; terms in insurance processing, anatomy and physiology, law, ethics; terms in surgical procedures, common diseases, common pathology
Pharmacology	10%–12.5%	PDR; basic drug calculation, metric conversions; terms and abbreviations; prescription requirements, drug schedules, classes of drugs; common drugs, side effects, indications; Drug Enforcement Agency regulations; preparation and administration, routes, drug forms

CLIA, Clinical Laboratory Improvement Amendments; OSHA, Occupational Safety and Health Administration; PDR, Physicians' Desk Reference.

Content Outline of NCMOA Examination

Knowledge Area	Approx. % of Exam	Topics
Insurance	20%	Managed-care models, third-party payers; types of insurance plans, filing claims; referrals and precertification; DRGs, basic procedure and diagnostic coding
Law and ethics	22%	Legal terms; confidentiality and HIPAA; professionalism and ethics
Medical terminology	31%	Word structure; pharmaceutical and medical abbreviations and symbols; terms in insurance processing, common diseases, and pathology; terms in surgical procedures, common diseases, and pathology
Office procedures	27%	Verbal and written communication; supplies, equipment; medical records; appointment and scheduling maintenance; basic financial management; basic health history interview, charting, vital signs, examination preparation; office emergencies, safety; understanding scope of practice

DRGs, diagnosis-related groups; HIPAA, Health Insurance Portability and Accountability Act.

AMCA National Examinations to Earn MAAC/MAC/CMAC Credentials

- Examinations are timed.
- Each examination question has 4 choices to select from (A through D).
- The MAAC examination consists of 240 questions; the MAC examination consists of 100 questions; the CMAC examination consists of 200 questions.

- Each question is weighted in value (1/4 point to 1 full point).
- A minimum score of 70 is required to pass each of these examinations.
- Applicants will know immediately on completion of the computerized examination whether they have earned the MAAC/MAC//CMAC credential.

Content Outline of MAAC Examination

Knowledge Area	% of Exam	# of Items
HIPAA and Compliance	19%	19
Scheduling	13%	13
Medical Records	11%	11
Other Administrative Knowledge	9%	9
Medical Terminology and Anatomy	13%	13
Emergency Care	9%	9
Medical Billing and Coding	11%	11
Insurance	15%	15

From http://www.AMCAexams.com.

Content Outline of MAC Examination

Knowledge Area	% of Exam	# of Items
Health-care systems	13%	13
Safety/Infection Control	17%	17
Anatomy and Physiology	15%	15
Medical Office Administrative	17%	17
Patient Care	19%	19
Medical Law and Ethics	19%	19

From http://www.AMCAexams.com.

Content Outline of CMAC Examination

Knowledge Area	% of Exam	# of Items
Anatomy and Physiology	12%	24
Phlebotomy	25%	50
ECG	11%	22
OSHA/Infection Control	19.5%	39
Medical Law and Ethics	11%	22
Medical Office/Patient Care Skills	14.5%	29
Health-care Systems	7%	14

From http://www.AMCAexams.com.

Maintaining Your Certification

From the AMT (RMA and CMAS)

- Pay an annual fee ($50), and every 3 years demonstrate activities supporting AMT certification.
- Earn 30 CEUs every 3 years through:
  - Satisfactory employment in the field (verified satisfactory and competent recent work history)
  - Traditional continuing education (AMT webinar, *AMT Journal of Continuing Education*)
  - Formal education (earned college, junior college credits in related field)
  - Professional education (state and/or national conventions, seminars and/or training; all need to be in related field)
  - Authoring written works (must be related to certification field)
  - Instructional presentations (prepared and presented related to employment and/or certification
- Track your CEUs online.

From the AAMA (CMA)

- Pay an annual fee, and every 5 years demonstrate activities supporting AAMA certification.
- Earn 60 CEUs every 5 years. The AAMA requires that a minimum of 30 CEUs be from the AAMA and earned in the following competency areas:
  - 10 must be from general.
  - 10 must be from clinical.
  - 10 must be from administrative.
  - The remaining 30 may be from any combination of the foregoing categories.
- Ways to earn the required CEUs are:
  - Continuing education (CMA journal, e-learning center articles, AAMA self-study courses)
  - Professional education (AAMA local chapter, state and/or national conventions or other approved education)
  - Formal education (earned college, junior college credits in related field)
- Track your CEUs online.

From the NCCT (NCMA or NCMOA)

- Pay an annual fee, and earn 14 CEUs each year to maintain an active credential.
- Ways to earn the required CEUs are as follows:
  - Online free CEUs may be earned by members on the NCCT website.
  - Paper coursework may be downloaded from the NCCT website.
  - CEUs can be earned by formal education (college, junior college credits in related field).
  - NCCT offers live webinars for CEU credits; go online to ncctinc.com and select "stay certified" or call customer service at 1-800-875-4404.
  - Contact the NCCT for other opportunities to earn CEUs.

From the AMCA (MAAC or MAC or CMAC)

- There is no annual fee required to maintain an active credential.
- Earn 10 CEUs every 2 years through:
  - Available CE volumes or the AMCA's Career Advancement Certificate Programs (volumes are worth 5 credits each)
  - Visiting MedlineUniversity.com for free continuing education
  - Satisfactory employment in the field (verified satisfactory and competent recent work history)
  - Traditional continuing education (publications or webinars from accredited medical assisting associations)
  - Formal education (earned college and/or junior college credits in related field)
  - Professional education (acquired from state conventions, national conventions, seminars, and/or training; all need to be in related field)
  - Authoring written works (must be related to certification field)
  - Instructional presentations (prepared and presented related to employment and/or certification)
- Track your CEUs online.

Study Plan Forms

Use the following forms to help you create and track a study plan for this book. See following pages.

Examination Preparation Progress Record

Use this log to keep track of your progress toward examination readiness.

Suggested Keys for Marking Mastery Level

No mark = Not yet studied
M = Mastered (100% correct)
K = Knowledgeable (80% or more correct)
P = Passing grade (75% correct)
I = Improvement needed (60% or less correct)

Examination Study Plan/Record Chapter 2

Examination Date: _____

Week of _____ (circle one) Study: First Second Third Fourth Fifth Sixth Last Again

Subject Area	Monday	Tuesday	Wednesday	Thursday	Friday	Saturday	Sunday
Medical Law and Ethics	Read	Reviewed	Quizzed			Reviewed again	

Examination Study Plan/Record Chapter 3

Examination Date: _____

Week of _____ (circle one) Study: First Second Third Fourth Fifth Sixth Last Again

Subject Area	Monday	Tuesday	Wednesday	Thursday	Friday	Saturday	Sunday
Anatomy, Physiology, and Medical Terminology	Read	Reviewed	Quizzed			Reviewed again	

Examination Study Plan/Record Chapter 4

Examination Date: _____

Week of _____ (circle one) Study: First Second Third Fourth Fifth Sixth Last Again

Subject Area	Monday	Tuesday	Wednesday	Thursday	Friday	Saturday	Sunday
Psychology and Interpersonal Communication	Read	Reviewed	Quizzed			Reviewed again	

Examination Study Plan/Record Chapter 5

Examination Date: _____

Week of _____ (circle one) Study: First   Second   Third   Fourth   Fifth   Sixth   Last   Again

Subject Area	Monday	Tuesday	Wednesday	Thursday	Friday	Saturday	Sunday
Medical Office Administration	Read	Reviewed	Quizzed			Reviewed again	

Examination Study Plan/Record Chapter 6

Examination Date: _____

Week of _____ (circle one) Study: First Second Third Fourth Fifth Sixth Last Again

Subject Area	Monday	Tuesday	Wednesday	Thursday	Friday	Saturday	Sunday
Medical Insurance, Billing, and Coding	Read	Reviewed	Quizzed			Reviewed again	

Examination Study Plan/Record Chapter 7

Examination Date: _____

Week of _____ (circle one) Study: First   Second   Third   Fourth   Fifth   Sixth   Last   Again

Subject Area	Monday	Tuesday	Wednesday	Thursday	Friday	Saturday	Sunday
Medical Office Communication	Read	Reviewed	Quizzed			Reviewed again	

Examination Study Plan/Record Chapter 8

Examination Date: _____

Week of _____ (circle one) Study: First Second Third Fourth Fifth Sixth Last Again

Subject Area	Monday	Tuesday	Wednesday	Thursday	Friday	Saturday	Sunday
Clinical Skills	Read	Reviewed	Quizzed			Reviewed again	

Examination Study Plan/Record Chapter 9

Examination Date: _____

Week of _____ (circle one) Study: First Second Third Fourth Fifth Sixth Last Again

Subject Area	Monday	Tuesday	Wednesday	Thursday	Friday	Saturday	Sunday
Pharmacology	Read	Reviewed	Quizzed			Reviewed again	

Examination Study Plan/Record Chapter 10

Examination Date: _____

Week of _____ (circle one) Study: First Second Third Fourth Fifth Sixth Last Again

Subject Area	Monday	Tuesday	Wednesday	Thursday	Friday	Saturday	Sunday
Laboratory Diagnostics	Read	Reviewed	Quizzed			Reviewed again	

Chapter 2: Medical Law and Ethics	Mastery Level	Self-Test Scores			
Subject Area		1	2	3	4

Chapter 3: Anatomy, Physiology, and Medical Terminology	Mastery Level	Self-Test Scores			
Subject Area		1	2	3	4

Chapter 4: Psychology and Interpersonal Communication	Mastery Level	Self-Test Scores			
Subject Area		1	2	3	4

Chapter 5: Medical Office Administration	Mastery Level	Self-Test Scores			
Subject Area		1	2	3	4

Chapter 6: Medical Insurance, Billing, and Coding	Mastery Level	Self-Test Scores			
Subject Area		1	2	3	4

Chapter 7: Medical Office Communications	Mastery Level	Self-Test Scores			
Subject Area		1	2	3	4

Chapter 8: Clinical Skills	Mastery Level	Self-Test Scores			
Subject Area		1	2	3	4

Chapter 9: Pharmacology	Mastery Level	Self-Test Scores			
Subject Area		1	2	3	4

Chapter 10: Laboratory Diagnostics	Mastery Level	Self-Test Scores			
Subject Area		1	2	3	4

Schedule Planner/Organizer Month _____

Sunday	Monday	Tuesday	Wednesday	Thursday	Friday	Saturday

YOUR NOTES

_____

_____

_____

_____

_____

_____

_____

Chapter 2
Medical Law and Ethics

Law is the system of rules regulating the behavior of people in a society. Law is beneficial to a society and enforces penalties for violation of those rules and standards. Ethics is the moral belief of what is valuable to us and determines how we conduct our lives. It addresses the moral standards and principles in our individual lives that determine right and wrong. To behave in an ethical manner is to understand that we all have choices that affect our well-being and those around us. Good decision-making is based on our knowledge of what is right and what is wrong.

Therefore, this chapter begins with a review of the types of law and their main areas, along with their related legal terms. Emphasis is placed on the types of civil law: tort, contract, administrative. Other sections recap the types of ambulatory health-care employee credentials available, the forms of medical practices, and the federal laws and acts related to health care. The last sections cover the area of ethics and include copies of the Standards of Practice of the American Medical Technologists (AMT), the Code of Ethics of the American Association of Medical Assistants (AAMA), and the Code of Ethics of the American Medical Certification Association (AMCA).

Information regarding medical law and ethics content within the various national certifying exams may be found in Chapter 1.

Remember to use Edge after you finish this chapter to test your knowledge. Directions for how to access Edge, as well as your access code, are located on the inside front cover of this text.

Law

Law comprises society's mandated rules and governmental punishment for failure to observe those rules.

Source of Law: 3 Branches of Government

- **Legislative (Congress):** Passes law.
- **Executive:** Administers law.
- **Judicial:** Interprets and enforces law.

Study Tip

For each term, highlight, underline, or otherwise mark 1 to 4 key words within each definition to help you memorize the term. See the 1st 2 terms below for examples.

Main Areas of Law

- **Criminal:** Crimes committed against society, an individual, or property. The government prosecutes the defendant, and if the defendant is found guilty, the result is imprisonment or fine.
- **Civil** (tort and/or contract): Concerns disputes or alleged wrongs committed against an individual or property by an individual or organization. The individual or group prosecutes, and if the defendant is found guilty, the result is monetary compensation.

Types of Civil Law

Tort

A tort is an accidental or intentional wrongful act by someone against another person or against property.

Negligence (most common tort): Failure to perform professional duties prudently, according to the accepted standard of care.

The forms of negligence include the following:

- **Nonfeasance:** Failure to act when duty is indicated; results in injury to another.
- **Misfeasance:** Improper performance of an act; results in injury to another.

- **Malfeasance:** Committing an improper (illegal) act; results in injury to another.
- **Malpractice** ("professional negligence"): Professional misconduct, lack of skill, wrongful practice; results in injury to another.
  - *Res ipsa loquitur* ("The thing speaks for itself"): Negligence is obvious, and the event could not have occurred without negligence.
  - *Respondeat superior* ("Let the master answer"): The provider may not be directly responsible but is responsible for negligence of employees.
  - The "4 Ds" of malpractice:
    Duty: The provider and patient relationship was established.
    Dereliction: The provider neglected a professional obligation to act or acted improperly.
    Direct cause: Negative outcome is a direct result of the provider's actions or failure to act.
    Damages: A negative act resulted in the patient sustaining harm.

Contract

A contract is a voluntary agreement between 2 parties that creates enforceable obligations and rights.

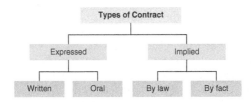

Types of Contract

Express contract: An agreement between 2 parties that details the responsibilities of both parties, written or oral. If written, it is signed by both parties.

Examples of health-care express contracts include the following:

- The Truth in Lending Act: This is a contract between the provider of care and the patient. It addresses scheduled payments to be made to the provider by the patient (most common when a large sum of money is owed for service).
- Medical Assistant Employment: This contract includes employee and employer duties, changes in job responsibilities, compensations, benefits, grievance procedures, terms of contract termination, termination procedures, and other special provisions.

Implied contract: The most common contract between providers and patients; not written, the result of actions (provider treats a patient within the physician's scope of practice).

Examples:

- The patient pays for provided services.
- An unconscious patient is treated in the emergency room.

Quid pro quo: Something for something.

- Service is rendered for payment.

Consent: An agreement between legally capable parties, legal intent is made; an offer is made and accepted, and transaction (service, payment) is made.

- **Consenter:** This can be a competent adult, emancipated minor (less than 18 years old), minor in the armed forces, minor parent with custody, or minor seeking sexually related treatment.
- **Informed consent:** Patient's right to know before agreeing to treatment, procedures, and care. Information disclosed to patients before treatment includes the potential benefits and risks of receiving and not receiving the treatment, as well as alternatives. The American Medical Association (AMA) suggests obtaining this beginning at the age of 15 years.
- **Uninformed consent:** Patient gives permission without full understanding.

Advance directive: Document states patient's wishes should he or she become incapable of making competent decisions; signed and witnessed.

Living will: Documentation of a patient's wish not to have certain life-sustaining measures taken when prognosis is imminent death.

Durable power of attorney (health care): Document allowing a designated person to act on behalf of patient to determine use of heroic or extraordinary measures.

Do not resuscitate order (DNR): Order originating from the patient as a directive to the health-care provider to withhold cardiopulmonary resuscitation if the patient experiences cardiac or respiratory arrest.

Administrative

Administrative law comprises government agency–enforced requirements and standards. Some agencies related to medical office operations are as follows:

- **Occupational Safety and Health Administration (OSHA):** A division of the U.S. Department of Labor, OSHA has jurisdiction over or administers the federal laws regulating safety in the workplace for employees and patients. A medical facility must be in compliance for controlling workers' exposure to infectious diseases through employee education and training in areas such as protective gear, decontamination, sharp equipment, laundry, exposure incidents, postexposure incidents, documentation, and hazardous materials. OSHA may conduct unannounced or complaint-response site inspections. If a site is not in compliance, the degree of penalty will depend on the severity of the offense.
  - **Bloodborne Pathogens Standard:** Protocols to protect from hepatitis B and C and from HIV; effective in 1991.
  - **Needlestick Safety and Prevention Act:** Promotes use of safer needles; identifies and documents devices used to ensure safety and new equipment monitoring; effective in 2003.

- **Hazard Communication Standard (HCS):** Sites must have a hazard plan for accidental exposure; manufacturers and chemical importers must provide material safety data sheet (MSDS) information and container labels.
- **Centers for Medicare & Medicaid Services (CMS):** This division of the U.S. Department of Health and Human Services (HHS) is the regulating agency for the **Clinical Laboratory Improvement Amendments (CLIA).** The HHS developed these federal regulations in 1988 to set standards for quality assurance performed in a laboratory and the accuracy of test results in the United States. The **Office of Clinical Standards and Quality (OCSQ)** has the responsibility of implementing and monitoring laboratory compliance with the CLIA regulations. The **Food and Drug Administration (FDA)** has the responsibility of determining the CLIA categorization of a laboratory test. The 3 CLIA regulatory categories of tests are as follows:
  - Waived tests: Simple, easy-to-perform procedures with a low risk of unreliable test results (includes FDA-approved at-home testing). A physician's office laboratory (POL) holding a certificate of waiver (CW) must adhere to good laboratory practice, including quality control of testing components, specimen handling, performance, and test results. Medical assistants may perform these tests.
  - Moderate-complexity tests: Not waived. Constitutes 75% of U.S. testing, most of which is performed by outside laboratories. Examples include microscopic examination of urine sediment, blood and urine cultures, and some blood chemistry studies. Testing personnel must meet education requirements higher than medical assisting.
  - High-complexity tests: Any procedure related to cytology (Pap testing), histopathology (tissue disease), cytogenetics (cell growth and origin), or histocompatibility (tissue matching). Education of personnel at this level is the most rigorous.

- **Internal Revenue Service (IRS):** Regulates payroll taxes.
- **Drug Enforcement Administration (DEA):** Regulates provider registration and all handling of controlled substances (i.e., medications) in the office.

YOUR NOTES

_____

_____

_____

_____

_____

_____

_____

Related Legal Terms and Definitions

Abandonment: Ceasing to care for or attend to a patient while the patient needs care. May be charged by the patient if the physician withdraws from the contractual relationship without notifying the patient while the patient still needs treatment.

Accreditation: Formal recognition that a facility meets predetermined standards for policies, practices, performance, and procedures. An outside agency grants accreditation after an on-site evaluation and survey and a self-study survey by the facility.

Affidavit: A verbal or written voluntary statement sworn to be true under oath before an authorized official.

Appellant: The party appealing the decision of a lower court to the jurisdiction of a higher court.

Arbitration: A dispute between parties that is settled by the judgment of an uninvolved 3rd-party person (or group) mutually selected by disputing parties.

Assault: A threat that is made with the capability of doing physical harm.

Battery: Nonconsensual touching of a person, without a legally justifiable reason, that is considered to be harmful or offensive; an intentional tort.

Common law ("Judge-made law"): Traditional laws based on earlier cases (precedents). The decisions are made by judges (courts) and take into account case-specific information. Because new precedents may be established, the principles of these cases continue to evolve. Settlers from England brought these laws with them.

Confidentiality: The expectation that when entrusting an individual with private information, it will remain private between the 2 involved parties. Confidentiality is a major ethical area of concern for all health-care professionals. Information is gained as a result of the physician-patient relationship. It is also referred to as privileged communication.

Defamation: False, malicious communication to a 3rd party; works to damage a person's reputation; includes libel and slander.

Defendant: The party against whom action (i.e., lawsuit) is being brought.

Emancipated minor: A person less than 18 years old who is responsible for their own debts.

Guardian: The individual assigned by the court to protect and make decisions on behalf of an individual who is not capable of making competent decisions.

In loco parentis: Status of person(s) assigned by the court system to represent the parent(s) in the legal rights, responsibilities, and duties toward a child. This is a legal doctrine.

Liability: Refers to damages resulting from a negligent act in which someone is directly responsible.

Libel: Deliberately defamatory written communication.

Medical record: A document containing the administrative and clinical information of a patient seen within a medical practice. The record may be in hard copy (paper) or in a digital format—only medical staff may have access to these records. Maintaining the medical record is a component of professional work ethic.

Moral: Concerned with ideas about right and wrong.

Plaintiff: The party bringing the suit or claim to court.

Protected health information (PHI): A patient's identifiable health information that may be transmitted or maintained by electronic or other media (e.g., faxes).

Privacy rule: In place to protect all PHI transferred, held, or transmitted by a covered entity.

Public law: The laws regulating the public at large: the rights and responsibilities of government to its citizens and vice versa.

Res judicata: Principle meaning once a case is resolved on its merits, it cannot be tried again on the basis of the same evidence.

Slander: Defamatory verbal communication.

Standard of care: Care given by a sound and rational person in the same situation; the measure against which a defendant's conduct is compared.

Stare decisis ("Let the decision stand"): Adherence to precedents made in cases that have already been decided.

Statute of limitations: Time limits for starting legal actions after a wrongful act, injury, or breach of contract occurs. The limitations vary from state to state. Factors influencing the limitations are as follows:

- Date contract ceased to exist between parties (patient and physician)
- Date of the wrongful act
- Date the physician terminated treatment
- Date the injury was discovered
- Date the discovery of the injury should have been made (reasonably)

Subpoena duces tecum: Commands an individual to appear in court with a patient's medical record or other pertinent documents.

Ambulatory Health-Care Employee Credentials

To be awarded a credential, an ambulatory health-care employee must pass an examination given by the state or other accrediting agency. The credentials bestowed on these individuals entitle them to authority and confidence in their field of education.

Licensed

Licenses are granted by individual states on meeting requirements to practice legally within the scope of the field. The applicant must pass the licensing examination and pay the license fee.

- **Licensed medical practitioners** (subject to the highest amount of regulation):
  - Medical doctors (MDs)
  - Doctors of osteopathy (DOs)
  - Registered nurses (RNs)
  - Licensed practical nurses (LPNs)
  - Licensed vocational nurses (LVNs)
- **Reciprocity:** License to practice granted when 1 state recognizes and accepts another state's licensing procedure.
- **License revocation or suspension**
  - Convicted of a crime
  - Guilty of unprofessional conduct (dishonesty, falsifying records)
  - Incapable professionally or personally (substance abuse, practicing outside trained scope)

Certified

Certification is granted by a professional organization on meeting its requirements. The applicant must pass the credentialing examination and pay the certification fee. The examination is usually for national certification.

- **Credentialed professions**
  - Certified as a Certified Medical Assistant (CMA)— Through the AAMA
  - Certified as a Registered Medical Assistant (RMA)— Through the AMT
  - Certified as a Medical Assistant National Certified Medical Assistant (MA NCMA)—Through the National Center for Competency Testing (NCCT)
  - Certified as a Certified Medical Administrative Specialist (CMAS)—Through the AMT
  - Certified as a National Certified Medical Office Assistant (NCMOA)—Through the NCCT
  - Certified as a Medical Administrative Assistant Certified (MAAC)—Through the AMCA
  - Certified as a Medical Assistant Certified (MAC)— Through the AMCA
  - Certified as a Clinical Medical Assistant (CMAC)— Through the AMCA
  - Medical Laboratory Technician (MLT)
  - Medical Technologist (MT)
  - Certified Medical Transcriptionist (CMT)
  - Certified Coding Associate (CCA)
  - Certified Coding Specialist (CCS)

Licensed and/or Certified

State regulation may require a license, certification, or both for nurse practitioners (NPs) and physician assistants (PAs).

Registration

On passing a credentialing examination that grants licensure or certification in a health field, the individual is registered with the field's professional organization (e.g., the AMT, AAMA, NCCT, or AMCA for medical assistants). To remain registered with the professional organization, the credentialed individual usually must earn continuing education units (CEUs) and usually pay a fee to the accrediting agency each year to reregister.

YOUR NOTES

_____

_____

_____

_____

_____

_____

_____

Types of Medical Practice

Solo practice: One medical practitioner owns the practice, makes all decisions, and retains all profits, costs, and liabilities.

Partnership: Two medical practitioners own the practice through a written agreement. They share costs, liabilities, profits, and decision-making.

Group practice: Three or more providers share costs, profits, and decisions (usually primary care, 1 specialty, or a multispecialty group).

Professional service corporation: This organization comprises various professionals (e.g., 1 or more medical providers or lawyers). Benefits may include profit sharing and pensions, individual liability, and state law regulation.

Federal Acts and Laws

Affordable Care Act: Informally known as "Obamacare"; reforms the health-care system by providing the qualified consumer (income meeting federal poverty levels) with less expensive health insurance and access to quality health care.

Americans With Disabilities Act (ADA): Prohibits discrimination (with 15 or more employees) in employment practices, hiring, fringe benefits, leaves, and terminations. Public accommodations must be made in a facility's architecture and to practice policies.

Child Abuse Prevention and Treatment Act: The state mandates for all professionally trained personnel (e.g., physicians, medical assistants, teachers) working with children to report suspected child abuse and neglect.

Civil Rights Act: Governs all forms of discrimination among employees, supervisors, and employers.

CLIA: Quality and complexity level regulations for hospital, private, and POLs; laboratory levels are waived, moderately complex, or highly complex.

Controlled Substances Act: Controls the prescribing, dispensing, and administering of narcotic, stimulant, and other dangerous drugs that can be abused; managed by the DEA.

Consolidated Omnibus Budget Reconciliation Act (COBRA): Ensures workers who have lost health insurance coverage for themselves and their families the right to choose to continue with their plan or move to an alternative health insurance coverage.

Employee Retirement Income Security Act (ERISA): Protects and regulates employee pensions.

Equal Credit Opportunity Act: Ensures all patients are offered extended credit; denial of an offer must be based on inability-to-pay rationale.

Equal Employment Opportunity Act (EEOA): Prohibits inquiry on job applications of race, color, sex, religion, national origin, medical history, arrest records, and past substance abuse.

Fair Credit Billing Act: Establishes time limits in billing complaints—the patient has 60 days to complain; the medical facility has 90 days to respond.

Fair Debt Collections Practices Act: Regulates debt collection practice and eliminates unfair practice.

Fair Labor Standards Act: Regulates employee wages, pay records, overtime pay, and child labor.

Family and Medical Leave Act (FMLA): Allows unpaid leave without position loss up to 12 weeks in sites employing more than 50 persons.

- Reasons for leave can be birth or adoption of child, ill family member, or own illness.
- Applies if employed for 1 year.

Genetic Information Nondiscrimination Act (GINA): Prohibits discrimination on the basis of genetic information with respect to health insurance coverage and employment.

Wage Garnishment Law: Requires an employer to withhold the earnings of an individual for the court-ordered payment of a debt. The law sets a dollar limit that can be attached to a person's wages or property.

Freedom of Information Act: Law allowing full or partial disclosure of previously unreleased information and documents controlled by the U.S. government. The act:

- Defines agency records subject to disclosure.
- Outlines mandatory disclosure.
- Grants 9 exemptions to the statute (confidential information).

Many state acts may be similar but not identical to the federal act.

Good Samaritan Law: Protects individuals stopping to give aid in an emergency situation (i.e., health-care employee giving aid to nonpaying individuals outside place of employment). Protects care provider from civil lawsuit if the provider is not found to be grossly negligent in the given care.

Health Insurance Portability and Accountability Act (HIPAA): Provides national guidelines for health-care privacy protection. Employees must be trained in HIPAA law and in the policies and procedures of a health-care office. There are 2 main sections of the law:

- **Title I: Health-Care Portability**
  - Protects insurance coverage for employee job changes.
  - Ensures the same plan and coverage.
  - Limits use of exclusions for preexisting conditions.
- **Title II: Administrative Simplification:** Addresses fraud and abuse prevention, medical liability reform, and privacy of health information.
  - Standards are in place to protect medical records and other patient information.
  - Patients have more control over health information (access, inspect, copy their record; request amendment to their record; obtain record of disclosures made of their record; complain regarding violations of the regulations and the provider's own information policies).
  - Safeguards are in place to protect patients' records.
  - Distinction is made between public responsibility to disclose information and violation of patients' rights.
  - Civil and criminal penalties are imposed on violators.

Medical Practice Acts: Each state's statutes that govern the practice of medicine (education, licensing and renewals, and suspension and revocation of license).

Occupational Safety and Health Act (OSHA): Regulates employee safety from known hazards causing death or injury. Mandates that MSDSs on hazardous products at sites are available to employees.

Patient's Bill of Rights: American Hospital Association (AHA) statement guaranteeing patients certain rights (e.g., service, confidentiality, receipt of updated information regarding diagnosis, treatment, physical examination; receipt of all information regarding procedures, bill examination and understanding).

Patient Self-Determination Act: Requires written information regarding rights, medical decision-making, and execution of advance directives be provided by health-care worker.

Truth in Lending Act (Regulation Z): Signed agreement for full debt payment in more than 4 payments; agreement also stipulates applied or nonapplied finance charge.

Uniform Anatomical Gift Act: States that any living individual of sound mind who is more than 18 years of age may donate all or parts of their body after death into tissue bank placement, or transplant, or research.

- The physician who determines the time of death cannot participate in the removal or transplant procedures or use the body parts for research.
- The physician cannot be sued for accepting the body parts if the physician did so in good faith that the proper documents were in place.

YOUR NOTES

_____

_____

_____

_____

_____

_____

_____

Ethics

Ethics is more concerned with values and virtues than with facts. In the health-care setting, ethics is about doing the right thing for the patient, the provider of services, and the facility. Both an individual's vision of right and wrong (based on life experience) and a more worldwide vision of right and wrong are considered in ethical predicament decision-making.

Medical Ethics

- *Medical ethics* refers to moral conduct of people in medical professions.

- Every medical profession has a code of ethics.
- Medical ethics contributes to the well-being of the community.
- Because of their responsibility to society, medical professionals must remain current in their knowledge and skills.

The result(s) of failure to adhere to ethical standards are:

- Negative reputation
- Suspension of certification or license by licensing or certifying board
- Revocation of certification or license revocation by licensing or certifying board

The following AMT Standards of Practice for RMAs and CMASs, the AAMA Code of Ethics for CMAs, and the AMCA Code of Ethics for MAACs, MACs, and CMACs serve as examples of the professional expectations of these certifying agencies. All licensing and certifying agencies have their own codes of conduct.

American Medical Technologists Standards of Practice

I.   While engaged in the arts and sciences that constitute the practice of their profession, AMT professionals shall be dedicated to the provision of competent and compassionate service and shall always meet or exceed the applicable standard of care.

II. The AMT professional shall place the health and welfare of the patient above all else.

III. When performing clinical duties and procedures, the AMT professional shall act within the lawful limits of any applicable scope of practice, and when so required shall act under and in accordance with appropriate supervision by an attending physician, dentist, or other licensed practitioner.

IV. The AMT professional shall always respect the rights of patients and of fellow health-care providers, shall comply with all applicable laws and regulations governing the privacy and confidentiality of protected health-care information, and shall safeguard patient confidences unless legally authorized or compelled to divulge protected health-care information to an authorized individual, law enforcement officer, or other legal or governmental entity.

V. AMT professionals shall strive to increase their technical knowledge, shall continue to learn, and shall continue to apply and share scientific advances in their fields of professional specialization.

VI. The AMT professional shall respect the law and pledges to avoid dishonest, unethical, or illegal practices, breaches of fiduciary duty, or abuses of the position of trust into which the professional has been placed as a certified health-care professional.

VII. AMT professionals understand that they shall not make or offer a diagnosis or dispense medical advice unless they are duly licensed practitioners or unless specifically authorized to do so by an attending licensed practitioner acting in accordance with applicable law.

VIII. The AMT professional shall observe and value the judgment of the attending physician, dentist, or other attending licensed practitioner, provided that so doing does not clearly constitute a violation of law or pose an immediate threat to the welfare of the patient.

IX. AMT professionals recognize that they are responsible for any personal wrongdoing and that they have an obligation to report to the proper authorities any knowledge of professional abuse or unlawful behavior by any party involved in the patient's diagnosis, care, and treatment.

X. The AMT professional pledges to uphold personal honor and integrity and to cooperate in protecting and advancing, by every lawful means, the interests of the American Medical Technologists and its Members.

Reprinted with permission of the American Medical Technologists (www.americanmedtech.org).

American Association of Medical Assistants Code of Ethics

Members of AAMA dedicated to the conscientious pursuit of their profession, and thus desiring to merit the high regard of the entire medical profession and the respect of the general public which they serve, do pledge themselves to strive always to:

A. Render service with full respect for the dignity of humanity;
B. Respect confidential information obtained through employment unless legally authorized or required by responsible performance of duty to divulge such information;
C. Uphold the honor and high principles of the profession and accept its disciplines;
D. Seek to continually improve the knowledge and skills of medical assistants for the benefit of patients and professional colleagues;
E. Participate in additional service activities aimed toward improving the health and well-being of the community.

Reprinted with permission of the American Association of Medical Assistants (www.aama-ntl.org).

American Medical Certification Association Code of Ethics

The AMCA believes in a high code of moral ethics. Should you become certified by the AMCA, you must agree to abide by the following code of ethics:

1. Be dedicated to your profession. Participate actively in continuing education to enhance your knowledge of your profession.
2. Practice good judgment and be honest in all professional interactions.
3. Respect the rights of your clients and be consistently aware of HIPAA laws and how they apply to both you and your client.

4. Practice empathy toward your clients.
5. Support and respect state and federal mandates as they apply to your profession.
6. Report any wrongdoings to the appropriate personnel.

Bioethics

Bioethics is the moral inquiry into issues brought about by advances in medicine and biological science. It focuses particularly on ethical controversies brought about by current biomedical technology and research, which are often life-and-death moral issues.

Individuals make their own decisions; no laws govern their choice. These issues have no clear answers, and patients' decisions affect their lives.

YOUR NOTES

_____

_____

_____

_____

_____

_____

Sample Certification Test Questions

1. Which of the following prevents employers from discriminating against individuals on the basis of race, color, religion, sex, age, or national origin?
   A. Civil Rights Act
   B. Equal Employment Opportunity Act

C. Immigration Reform Act
D. Labor Management Relations Act
E. National Labor Relations Act

2. Physicians are legally obligated to do which of the following after a physician-patient contract has been established?

A. Bill the patient's insurance company for all services.
B. Evaluate the patient for any medical problem.
C. Release the patient's medical records when requested by telephone.
D. Treat the patient within the physician's scope of practice.
E. Write off differences between service charges and allowable amounts.

3. Which of the following statutes includes regulations regarding the testing of patient specimens and interpreting of results in the medical office?

A. Clinical Laboratories Improvement Amendments (CLIA 1988)
B. Controlled Substances Act
C. Food, Drug, and Cosmetic Act
D. Medical Practice Act
E. Occupational Safety and Health Act

See the Appendix for the answers.

DAVIS
edge.

Remember to use Edge after you finish this chapter to test your knowledge. Directions for how to access Edge, as well as your access code, are located on the inside front cover of this text.

Chapter 3

Anatomy, Physiology, and Medical Terminology

The science of anatomy concerns the structure of the body; the term *anatomy* comes from the Greek word meaning to dissect. Most medical terminology is Greek in origin. The science of physiology is concerned with how the body functions or works. The science of pathophysiology concerns any condition or disease resulting from the improper functioning of body parts.

This chapter begins with common medical terminology. Common prefixes, suffixes, and word roots are given here. This is followed by a review of basic human structure from atoms to body systems. This chapter will then touch upon a few notable diseases, epidemics, and/or pandemics that have affected more than 1 body system and have frequently been deadly in recent years before delving into the individual body systems.. The chapter covers each body system in 12 sections. Each section gives you the anatomy, physiology, common tests performed, and various conditions and diseases associated with the system. At the end of each body system, you will find a list of word roots specific to that system.

Information regarding anatomy, physiology, and medical terminology content within the various national certifying exams may be found in Chapter 1.

Remember to use Edge after you finish this chapter to test your knowledge. Directions for how to access Edge, as well as your access code, are located on the inside front cover of this text.

Directional Terminology

Term	Definition	Example of Usage
Left (L)	L side of patient's body	Stomach is to L of liver
Right (R)	R side of patient's body	"The R kidney is damaged."
Superior	Toward top of body	Shoulders are superior to hips
Inferior	Toward lower end of body	Stomach is inferior to heart
Anterior/ventral	Toward front of body	Nose is on anterior of head
Posterior/dorsal	Toward back of body	Vertebral column is posterior to sternum
A&P	Anterior and posterior; or auscultation and percussion	The frontal plane divides the body into anterior and posterior portions
		Auscultation and percussion are used to assess the lungs
Caudad (caudal)	Toward tail	Neck is caudad to skull
Cephalad	Toward head	Neck is cephalad to tail
Medial	Toward midsagittal; away from side	Eyes are medial to ears
Lateral	Toward side; away from midsagittal	Eyes are lateral to nose

Directional Terminology—cont'd		
Term	Definition	Example of Usage
Distal	Away from point of origin; from the trunk or point of attachment	Hand is distal to elbow
Proximal	Closest to point of origin, toward trunk (position in a limb or appendage)	Joint is proximal to toenail
Visceral	Toward internal organ; away from outer wall	Organ covered with visceral layer of the membrane
Parietal	Toward wall; away from internal structures	Abdominal cavity lined with parietal peritoneal membranes
Deep	Toward inside of part; away from surface	Thigh muscles deep to skin
Superficial	Toward surface of part; away from inside	Skin is a superficial organ
Medullary	Refers to an inner region, or medulla	Medullary portion of organ contains nerve tissue
Cortical	Refers to an outer region or cortex	Cortical area produces hormones

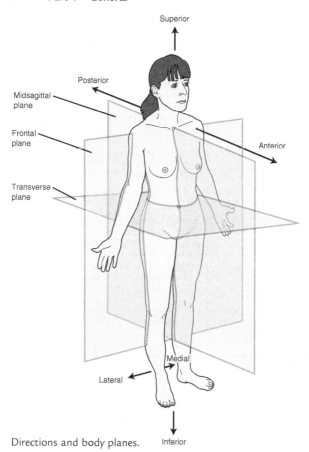

Directions and body planes.

Movement Terminology

Adduction: State of drawing toward the middle.

Abduction: State of drawing away from the middle.

Afferent: Movement toward the center (core). Afferent nerves carry information to the central nervous system (CNS) from the peripheral nervous system (PNS).

Circumduction: Drawing an imaginary circle with a body part (e.g., finger or arm movement).

Efferent: Movement away from the center. Efferent nerves carry information away from the CNS to muscles and glands.

Eversion: State of turning outward (turning wrists and ankles outward, away from the body).

Extension: Movement of a limb into a straight position (straightening the fingers of the hand).

Flexion: Movement in which a limb is bent (bringing the hand up to touch the shoulder).

Inversion: State of turning inward.

Plantar flexion: Pointing the toes downward.

Prone: Lying straight on one's front side; face down.

Rotation: Turning on an axis (head turning from side to side).

Supine: Lying straight on one's back, face up.

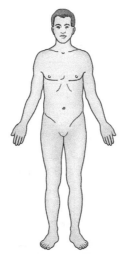

Anatomical position; palms front.

Text continued on page 66

Common Prefixes			
Prefix	Common Meaning	Prefix	Common Meaning
a, an	Without or absence of	hypo	Deficient, decreased
ab	Away from	inter	Between, among
ad, af, ap, as, at	Toward, in the direction of	intra	Within, inside
ana	Excessive	meta	Change, after, beyond
bi	2, life	neo	New
bin	2 by 2	nulli	None
brady	Slow	pan	All, total
dia	Through, complete	para	Beside, beyond, around
dipl	Double, twin	per	Through
dys	Bad, difficult, painful	peri	Surrounding
endo	Within	poly	Many
epi	On	post	After
eti	Cause	pre	Before
eu	Good, normal, well, easy	sub	Under, less, below
ex, exo	Outside, outward	super, supra	Above, excessive
hemi	Half	syn, sym	Together, joined
hyper	Excessive, increased	tachy	Fast, rapid

Common Suffixes			
Suffix	Common Meaning	Suffix	Common Meaning
ectasis	Stretching out, dilation, expansion	ical, ial, ic, ior	Pertaining to
ectomy	Surgical removal	ictal	Seizure, attack
emia	Blood condition	itis	Inflammation
emesis	Vomiting	lysis	Loosening, dissolution, separating
gen	Agent that causes or produces	malacia	Abnormal softening
genesis	Origin, cause	megaly	Enlargement
genic	Producing, causing, originating	meter	Instrument used to measure
gram	An instrument for recording, picture, record	metry	Measurement
graphy	Process of producing a picture	necrosis	Tissue death
ia	Diseased, abnormal condition	odynea	Pain
iasis, esis	Condition	oid	Resembling
iatry	Physician, treatment	ologist	Specialist
ology	The study of	physis	Growth
oma	Tumor	plasia	Formation

Continued

Common Suffixes—cont'd

Suffix	Common Meaning	Suffix	Common Meaning
opia	Vision	plasm	Formative material of cells
opsy	To view	plasty	Surgical repair
ory, ose, ous	Pertaining to	plegia	Paralysis
osis	Abnormal condition	pnea	Breathing
ostomy	Surgically created opening	poiesis	Formation
otomy	Surgical incision	ptosis	Drooping, sagging, prolapse
oxia	Oxygen	rrhage, rrhagia	Bleeding, bursting forth
paresis	Slight paralysis	rrhaphy	Surgical suturing
pathy	Disease	rrhea	Flow, discharge
penia	Abnormal reduction in number	rrhexis	Rupture
pepsia	Digestion	sarcoma	Malignant tumor
pexy	Surgical fixation, suspension	schisis	Split, fissure
phagia	Eating, swallowing	scope	Visual exam with instrument
phobia	Abnormal fear or aversion to	scopy	Visual examination
phonia	Sound, voice	sis	State of

Common Suffixes—cont'd

Suffix	Common Meaning	Suffix	Common Meaning
spasm	Sudden involuntary muscle contraction	tripsy	Surgical crushing
stasis	Control, maintenance at a constant level	trophy	Development
stenosis	Abnormal tightening, narrowing	thorax	Chest
tome	Instrument used to cut	uria	Urine, urination

Common Word Roots

Root	Meaning	Root	Meaning
carcin	Cancer	melan	Black
chrom	Color	neur	Nerve
cyan	Blue	onc	Tumor
cyt	Cell	organ	Organ
erythr	Red	path	Disease
gno	Knowledge	rhabd	Rod-shaped or striated (tissue)
hist	Tissue	sarc	Flesh, connective tissue
kary	Nucleus	somat	Body
lei	Smooth	viscer	Internal organs
leuk	White	xanth	Yellow
lip	Fat		

Body Structure

Body Cavities

Cranial
(brain)

Thoracic
(heart, lungs, large blood
vessels, separated from
abdomen by *diaphragm*)

Spinal
(spinal cord)

Abdominal
(stomach, most of intestines,
kidneys, liver, gallbladder,
pancreas, spleen, separated
from thoracic by diaphragm
and from pelvic by imaginary
line across top of hip bones)

Pelvic
(bladder, rectum,
reproductive organs)

Body cavities.

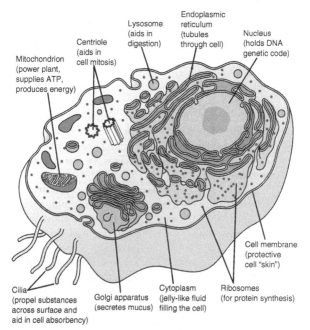

The cell.

Organization

Atom: This is the smallest chemical unit of matter.

Molecule: A combination of 2 or more atoms that together make the smallest unit of a substance. An element or compound can be a substance. The water molecule (H_2O) is made up of 2 hydrogen atoms and 1 oxygen atom.

Cell: This basic unit of life is the building block for tissues, organs, and so forth.

- Cell division
  - **Mitosis:** The division of 1 cell into 2 identical cells
  - **Meiosis:** The division of sex cells for organisms that sexually reproduce

- Cell actions
  - **Active transport:** The movement of molecules from an area of high concentration to low concentration. This is made possible because of adenosine triphosphate (ATP), a high-energy compound.
  - **Diffusion:** The passive movement of dissolved particles through a membrane from areas of high concentration to low concentration. Diffusion is the most common transport mechanism.
  - **Filtration:** The use of mechanical pressure to diffuse liquids through membranes. This is a form of passive transport.
  - **Osmosis:** A type of diffusion in which water or other selected substances in solution pass through a semipermeable membrane. The membrane allows some substances to pass through it but excludes others. This is a form of passive transport.
  - **Passive transport:** No cellular energy is required to move water and dissolved substances.
  - **Phagocytosis:** The ingestion and digestion of substances by phagocytic cells (e.g., white blood cell [WBC] neutrophils). This process requires cellular energy.

Tissue: This grouping of cells performs a specific function.

The 4 Types of Tissues		
Tissue Type	**Locations**	**Functions**
Epithelial	Skin, tubes, ducts, some glands, linings of cavities	Protection, absorption, secretions, excretions
Connective	Bones, cartilage, tendons, muscle sheaths, blood	Supports, connects other tissues and structures
Muscle	3 types: striated, smooth, cardiac	Produces movement, contracts or shortens
Nerve	Neurons (cells) throughout body	Actively transmits impulses through networks

Organ: An organ is a body structure made up of a group of tissues that serve a common purpose or function.

System: A group of organs that work together to perform a specific function. For example, the urinary system is made up of the following organs: kidneys, ureters, bladder, and urethra. This system cleanses the blood of waste products and provides a route for the waste (urine) to exit the body.

Homeostasis: Equilibrium, maintaining a balance of the internal body. The body strives to maintain this "healthy" state.

YOUR NOTES

_____

_____

_____

_____

_____

_____

Diseases, Epidemics, and Pandemics of Recent Concern

The World Health Organization (WHO) and the Centers for Disease Control and Prevention (CDC) continue to have concerns about the rise of new threats and those already known to us. The following is a brief description of the diseases, epidemics, and/or pandemics that have emerged in recent years.

Anthrax: Originated in Egypt and Mesopotamia. It is a rare but serious infection caused by a spore-forming bacterium.

It can occur in 4 forms: skin, lungs, intestinal, and injection. Humans become infected through contact with an infected animal or by inhaling spores. Symptoms range from a skin ulcer to difficulty breathing. Inhaled anthrax can be fatal because it is more difficult to treat. This infection is treatable with antibiotics.

***Candida auris* infection:** May be acquired in hospitals by patients with weakened immune systems. Caused by a species of fungus that grows as yeast in an open wound, the bloodstream, or the ear. Most *C. auris* infections are treatable with a class of antifungal drugs; however, some are resistant.

COVID-19 (coronavirus disease 2019 [SARS-COV 2]): In 2020 this became a pandemic. It is thought to have originated in China. It is not the same as the coronaviruses that commonly circulate among humans and cause mild illness, such as the common cold. It is highly contagious through respiratory droplets when in close contact with others and contaminated surfaces. Symptoms range from mild to severe and appear 2 to 14 days after exposure to the virus. Older adults and people with severe underlying medical conditions are at high risk for developing more serious complications and death. As of this writing there is no cure.

Ebola: Also known as **Ebola hemorrhagic fever (EHF)** or **Ebola virus disease (EVD):** Believed to be an animal-borne virus, likely from bats or apes. Originated in West Africa. Outbreaks occurred from 2014 to 2016. The virus spreads through contact with bodily fluids, animals, insects, and contaminated surfaces. Symptoms begin 2 days to 3 weeks after contracting the infection and cause severe bleeding and organ failure. It is often fatal, and there is no cure.

H1N1 influenza: It is a novel form of influenza A. It became a pandemic in 2009 and caused the 1918 flu pandemic. Originally referred to as **"swine flu."** It is actually a combination of viruses from pigs, birds, and humans. It was detected in the United States first and spread quickly across the United States and the world. It is highly contagious through contaminated droplets and surfaces. Upper and lower respiratory and gastrointestinal distress, fatigue, confusion, seizures, and fever are signs and symptoms. Symptoms begin 1 to 3 days after exposure. A vaccine has been approved. The virus is now known as H1N1v.

MRSA (methicillin-resistant *Staphylococcus aureus*): Referred to as a "super bug." It is the cause of staph infection that is difficult to treat because of resistance to some antibiotics. It can spread in hospitals, other health-care facilities, or where you live, work, and go to school. It is transmitted most often by direct skin-to-skin contact or contact with shared items or surfaces. It is a painful skin infection, a bump filled with pus accompanied by fever. Treatment for this is a course of antibiotic therapy over several days.

SARS (severe acute respiratory syndrome): Caused by a strain of coronavirus, the same family that causes the common cold. This virus is rare and first appeared in China. Scientists suspect the virus evolved from 1 or more animal viruses into a new strain. It is contagious and sometimes fatal. It spread worldwide; however, no known transmission has occurred anywhere in the world since 2004.

Zika virus disease: This disease was first discovered in 1947 and is named after the Zika forest in Uganda. It is similar to dengue fever, yellow fever, and West Nile virus. In 2016 the WHO declared it a pandemic. It is transmitted primarily by bites from infected *Aedes* mosquitoes. These mosquitoes bite during the day. The source of this disease is an infected animal, insect bite (such as a mosquito), or insect sting. In most cases there are no symptoms. Common symptoms are fever, rash, joint pain, and red eyes that usually last 2 to 7 days. In a few cases the disease can trigger birth defects in pregnant women. As of January 2020, there were no new areas of a current Zika outbreak. There is no vaccine or medication available to treat the disease.

Skeletal System

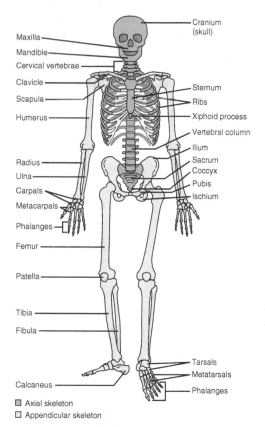

Maxilla

Mandible

Cervical vertebrae

Clavicle

Scapula

Humerus

Radius

Ulna

Carpals

Metacarpals

Phalanges

Femur

Patella

Tibia

Fibula

Calcaneus

Cranium
(skull)

Sternum

Ribs

Xiphoid process

Vertebral column

Ilium

Sacrum

Coccyx

Pubis

Ischium

Tarsals

Metatarsals

Phalanges

☐ Axial skeleton
☐ Appendicular skeleton

Skeletal system.

Structures and Functions of the Skeletal System	
Functions	**Cells, Tissues, Organs**
• Movement of body • Support of body (framework); gives us our basic shape • Attachment for muscle; gives muscle support • Formation of red blood cells in red bone marrow • Storage of calcium • Protection of internal organs	• Joints • Ligaments • Cartilage • Bone (approximately 206)

Organization

Axial Skeleton: The Major Bones	
Cranium (skull; seams are sutures)	**Frontal:** Forehead and eye sockets **Temporal:** Sides around ear and lower jaw **Parietal:** Sides above temporal and top **Occipital:** Back of head and skull base **Ethmoid:** Between nasal cavity and orbits **Sphenoid:** Supports nasal cavity
Facial (the major bones)	**Mandible:** Lower jaw **Maxilla:** Upper jaw **Zygomatic:** Arch of cheek; high portion (cheekbone) **Nasal:** Upper part of nose bridge **Palatine:** Hard palate of mouth and floor of nose
Smallest bones of the body	Malleus, incus, stapes (in the ear)
Column (spine; 26 bones)	Cervical: C1–C7, curve inward; C1, **atlas** (head movement for up-down); C2, **axis** (head movement side to side) Thoracic: T1–T12, curve outward Lumbar: L1–L5, curve inward Sacral: 5 fused vertebrae, curve out Coccyx: 4 fused vertebrae

Continued

Axial Skeleton: The Major Bones—cont'd	
Thorax (rib cage)	**Sternum:** Breastbone **(mediastinum)** • Xiphoid process: small, flat, bladelike bone tip at bottom of breastbone **Ribs:** 12 pairs

Appendicular Skeleton	
Upper extremities	**Humerus:** Upper arm, **largest arm bone** **Radius:** Lower arm, on thumb side **Ulna:** Lower arm, on little finger side **Carpals:** Wrist bones **Metacarpals:** Hand bones (palm) **Phalanges:** Fingers and thumb
Lower extremities	**Femur (thigh bone):** Largest, longest, strongest bone **Greater trochanter:** Knob at the top of the femur **Patella:** Kneecap **Tibia (shin bone):** Largest lower leg bone **Fibula:** Lower leg bone; on the lateral side of leg **Tarsals:** Ankle bones, the **calcaneus** (heel bone) is the largest of the tarsals **Metatarsals:** Foot bones **Phalanges:** Toe bones
Pectoral girdle	**Scapula (shoulder blade):** Upper back bone **Clavicle (collarbone):** Anterior shoulder bone
Pelvic girdle	**Ilium:** Winged-shaped portion **Ischium:** Inferior portion of hip; sit support **Pubis:** Anterior union of hip bones **Sacrum:** Posterior wall of the pelvis; 5 fused bones **Coccyx (tail bone):** 4 small fused vertebrae and ligaments

Joint Classifications

Synarthrosis (immovable): In these joints, 2 bones are separated only by a membrane (e.g., cranial sutures).

Amphiarthrosis (slightly movable): A fibrocartilaginous disk is located between 2 bones, or a ligament unites 2 bones (e.g., intervertebral disks).

Diarthrosis; synovial (freely movable): The ends of bones are joined by a joint capsule containing synovial fluid for lubrication:

- **Ball and socket (enarthrosis):** This joint allows the widest range of motion: flexion, extension, abduction, adduction, rotation, and circumduction (e.g., hips and shoulders).
- **Condyloid:** This joint allows all forms of angular movement except axial skeleton rotation (e.g., jaw).
- **Gliding (arthrodia):** This joint permits a single bony surface to slide on another, in a simple motion only (e.g., carpals).
- **Hinge (ginglymus):** This joint has only a single forward and backward motion: flexion or extension (e.g., elbow).
- **Pivot (trichoid):** This joint allows the rotation of bone (e.g., cervical spine C1 atlas [up and down] and C2 axis [side to side]).
- **Saddle:** In this joint, opposing surfaces are reciprocally concavo-convex: movement includes flexion, extension, abduction, adduction, and circumduction (e.g., thumb; carpometacarpal joint).

Additional Information

Bursa: A fibrous sac that acts as a cushion to ease movement

Condyle: A large, rounded knob that usually fits with another bone

Crest: A ridge on a bone

Foramen: A hole in bone serving as a passageway for vessels and/or nerves

Fossa: A depression or groove in a bone

Periosteum: A thick, fibrous membrane that covers a bone surface, except articular cartilage

Process: A prominent projection on a bone

Synovial fluid: A lubricating fluid for joints, bursae, and tendon sheaths to make smooth movement of a joint possible

Diagnostic Testing and Procedures

Arthrocentesis: A puncture performed to remove fluid for pressure pain relief or analysis

Arthroscopy: A procedure to view the internal structures of a joint and provide surgical access

Laminectomy with spinal fusion: A procedure to stabilize the vertebra by removing part of it

Traction and reduction: A procedure performed to realign the bones

X-ray: A radiograph of bones to examine for breaks or density

Common Diseases and Conditions

Cleft palate: A congenital deformity that occurs when the palatine bones have improperly closed. This leaves a passage between the mouth and the nasal cavities.

Fractures:

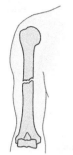

Closed, (simple)
(does not go through
the skin)

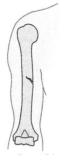

Greenstick
(incomplete)

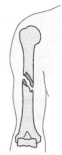

Spiral
(twisted break of bone)

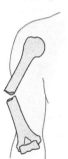

Compound, (open)
(complete break that
goes through the skin)

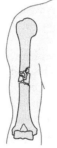

Comminuted
(bone is shattered into
3 or more fragments)

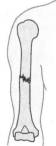

Impacted
(broken ends are forced
into one another)

Fractures.

Gout: Pain, usually in the great toe of the foot and possibly other body joints. This condition is brought on by a buildup of crystalizing uric acid resulting from high purine metabolism and other symptoms.

Kyphosis: An abnormal outward curvature of the spine (hunchback).

Lordosis: An abnormal inward curvature of the spine (swayback).

Osteoarthritis: An inflammation of the joints.

Osteomalacia: Softening and deformation of the bone are caused by vitamin D deficiency and result in a loss of calcium and phosphorus. It is known as **rickets** in children.

Osteoporosis: Bone mass reduction. Bones become thin, porous, and easily fractured.

Paget disease (osteitis deformans): Abnormal weakened bone formation is caused by excessive breakdown of bone tissue.

Phantom pain: A feeling of sensation in an absent, amputated limb.

Rheumatoid arthritis: An autoimmune disease causing painful and swelling joints resulting in deformities.

Scoliosis: A lateral, sideward curve of the spine.

Spondylosis: An inflammation of 1 or more vertebrae.

Sprain: An injury to a joint (wrist, ankle, knee), usually the result of a stretched or torn ligament.

Skeletal System Word Roots	
Root	Meaning
cost	Rib
arthr	Joint
ankyl	Crooked, stiff, bent
chondr	Cartilage
kinesi	Movement, motion
lamin	Lamina (thin, flat plate or layer)

YOUR NOTES

_____

_____

_____

_____

_____

_____

Muscular System

Structures and Functions of the Muscular System

Functions	Cells, Tissues, Organs

• Movement through cellular chemical reactions: muscle contracts and shortens and pulls a bone
• Maintains posture and alignment
• Protects bones and internal organs
• Generates heat
	• Muscles
	  • **Smooth (visceral):** Involuntary, within the walls of hollow organs; contractions cause movement **(peristalsis)**
	  • **Skeletal:** Voluntary, attached to bones; striated
	  • **Cardiac:** Involuntary, make up the walls of the heart; all cells work together for rhythmic cell pulse; striated
	• **Tendons:** Connective, attach muscle to periosteum of bone
	• **Ligaments:** Attach bone to bone (anterior cruciate of knee)

Organization

The body contains more than 600 muscles.

Examples of Muscles	
Muscle	**Location**
Biceps	Upper arm bender or flexor
Deltoid	Upper shoulder and arm (site for adult injections)
Gluteus medius	Buttocks, upper outer quadrant (injections at dorsogluteal or ventrogluteal site)
Masseter	Principal muscle in mastication
Pectoralis major	Chest
Triceps	Upper arm straightener or extensor
Vastus lateralis	Upper outer thigh (common site for infant injections)

See the diagram for more muscles and their locations.

Additional Information

Aponeurosis: A broad covering sheet of fibrous connective tissue that binds muscle to muscle or muscle to bone.

Diagnostic Testing and Procedures

Goniometry: Measures joint movement and angles.

Manipulation: This procedure examines range of motion; it is used in physical therapy.

Common Diseases and Conditions

Atrophy: Muscle wasting resulting from lack of use

Bursitis: An inflammation of the bursa (fluid-filled sac that reduces friction as joints move)

Cramp: A painful involuntary contraction by skeletal muscle

Epicondylitis: An inflammation of the forearm tendon (tennis elbow)

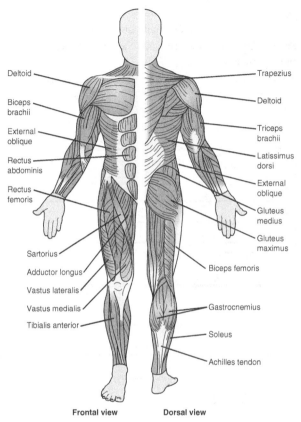

Frontal view   **Dorsal view**

Muscular system.

Fibromyalgia syndrome: A debilitating chronic condition characterized by specific or widespread muscle, bone, or joint pain, fatigue, and other symptoms

Muscular dystrophy: A genetic disease characterized by a wasting of skeletal muscles

Myasthenia gravis: An autoimmune neuromuscular disease caused by abnormal transmission of nerve impulses that results in muscle fiber atrophy or shrinkage, which inhibits normal movement, and extreme muscle weakness

Sprain: An injury in which ligaments around a joint are torn but not severed

Strain: Torn or overstretched (not severed) muscle or tear or overstretching at the attachment of a tendon (not at a joint location), usually caused by overuse

Tendonitis: An inflammation of tendons

Muscular System Word Roots	
Root	Meaning
bursa	Sac, cavity
fibr	Fibrous connective tissue
ten, tend, tendin	Tendon
my, myos	Muscle

YOUR NOTES

_____

_____

_____

_____

_____

_____

_____

Cardiovascular System

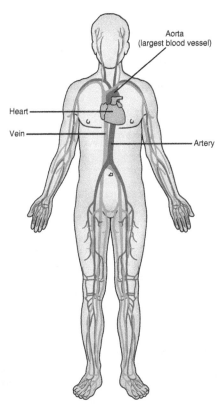

Cardiovascular system.

Structures and Functions of the Cardiovascular System	
Functions	**Cells, Tissues, Organs**

• Transports nutrients and oxygen to tissues
• Transports waste to organs for removal
• Assists in regulating body temperature
• Blood cells assist immune system (white blood cells)
• Assist in maintaining proper pH (O_2 and CO_2); normal blood pH is 7.35–7.45
	• Heart
	• Blood: 4–6 liters in normal adult
	  • 55% is plasma
	  • 45% is formed elements suspended in the plasma
	• Blood vessels

Organization

The cardiovascular system consists of the heart and blood vessels. They form a full circuit delivering oxygen (O_2)-rich blood for bodily function and ridding the body of waste byproducts (carbon dioxide [CO_2]) resulting from all body functions.

Heart

- The heart is located within the pericardium (a fluid-filled sac). The outer membrane of the sac is called the parietal pericardium; the inner membrane is called the visceral pericardium.
- The heart has 4 chambers: 2 upper atria (singular, atrium) and 2 lower ventricles. The left ventricle is larger and thicker.
- Blood passes through the hollow heart muscle. The heart muscle receives nourishment to function from the surrounding coronary arteries within the walls of the heart.

Interventricular septum: This wall of tissue divides the heart in half vertically.

Aortic semilunar valve: The valve that opens to allow O_2-rich blood to flow out of the left ventricle and into the aorta, which carries the blood to all parts of the body, except the lungs.

Mitral (bicuspid) valve: Closes the opening between the left atrium and the left ventricle to prevent backflow of O_2-rich blood back into the atrium once the blood has been pushed into the ventricle.

Pulmonary semilunar valve: The valve that opens to allow O_2-poor blood to flow out of the right ventricle and into the pulmonary artery, which carries the blood to the lungs.

Tricuspid valve: Closes the opening between the right atrium and the right ventricle to prevent backflow of O_2-poor blood back into the atrium once the blood has been pushed into the ventricle.

Arteries

- Arteries pulsate to transport blood away from heart and have the thickest-muscled vessel walls.
- They are rich with O_2 saturation. The only exception is the pulmonary artery, which exits the right side of the heart and transports CO_2 to the lungs.

Coronary artery: Supplies the blood needed for the cardiac muscles to function.

Aorta: Carrying the O_2-rich blood surging from the left ventricle of the heart, the aorta is the largest and thickest-walled artery in the body.

Carotid artery: Located on either side of the neck, this artery carries blood upward to the head. This is a common pulse site.

Brachial artery: Located on the inside of the elbow, this carries blood from the axillary artery to the radial and ulnar arteries. It is used for blood pressure (BP) reading.

Radial artery: Located on the thumb side of the wrist, it carries blood to the hand. It is the most commonly used pulse site.

Femoral artery: Located on the inner upper thigh, this artery carries blood from the inguinal ligament, branches, and then terminates at the popliteal artery. The femoral artery is used as a pulse site.

Arterioles: These downsized arteries have a thinner wall of muscle. They connect the arteries to the capillaries.

Veins

- Veins contain many valves to prevent blood backflow and transport blood to the heart.
- They have poor O_2 saturation. The only exception is the pulmonary vein, which enters the atrium on the left side of the heart with O_2-rich blood from the lungs.

Vena cava: This vein receives the blood from the upper (superior vena cava) and the lower (inferior vena cava) branches and transports it into the right atrium of the heart.

Median cubital, cephalic, and basilic veins: These veins drain blood from the forearm and hand, and they are the most commonly used veins for venipuncture. The most preferred site is the median cubital vein, the 2nd is the cephalic vein, and the 3rd is the basilic vein. All are located in the antecubital fossa (small depression inside the bend of the elbow and the forearm).

Venules: These small, thin veins connect the larger veins to the capillaries.

Capillaries

- Capillaries are 1 cell layer thick.
- They allow for the exchange of nutrients and waste products throughout the body.

Blood

- Blood is a type of connective tissue made up of cellular components and plasma. Its chief function is to transport nutrients and waste products to and from body tissues.

- Blood cellular components consist of red blood cells (RBCs), platelets, and white blood cells (WBCs).
  - **RBCs:** These biconcave cells have no nucleus and contain hemoglobin. They live 120 days and carry O_2 and CO_2. The average count is 5,000,000/mm^3 (5 million per cubic millimeter).
  - **Platelets:** These are also known as thrombocytes. They are cell fragments that help blood clot. The average count is 200,000/mm^3.
  - **WBCs:** There are 5 types to fight invading pathogens (infection). The average count is 5,000 to 10,000/mm^3. See Chapter 10 (Laboratory Diagnostics), hematology section for WBC type and function detail.
- Plasma is the liquid portion of blood in which cells are suspended.
- Most blood is formed in red bone marrow.

Diagnostic Testing and Procedures

Arteriogram: This test is an x-ray of the arteries.

BP reading: This diagnostic measurement is performed to determine the force of blood against artery walls.

Electrocardiogram (ECG): This is a printed tracing of a cardiac rhythm.

Stress test: This test measures heart activity during physical activity.

Pulse pressure: This is a measurement used by finding the difference between the systolic (maximum) and diastolic (minimum) BP readings.

Common Diseases and Conditions

Anemia: Abnormally low hemoglobin or RBCs in the bloodstream.

Angina pectoris: Severe chest pain caused by a low O_2 supply to the heart muscle. It may result from stress or activity.

Aneurysm: An outpouching of weakened blood vessel wall that may be caused by trauma or may be genetic.

Arteriosclerosis: A hardening, thickening, and loss of elasticity in the artery walls. The most common form of arteriosclerosis is atherosclerosis.

Atherosclerosis: A disease of the arteries caused by calcium and cholesterol plaque buildup on the artery walls, which restricts blood flow.

Bradycardia: A slow cardiac rhythm that is less than 60 beats per minute.

Congestive heart failure (CHF): This is a weakening of the heart's ability to pump blood effectively to meet the body's needs. This condition can cause pulmonary edema.

Claudication: A circulation problem of the arms and legs that points to a vascular disease. Symptoms are a limp and calf pain on walking that subsides at rest.

Heart block: The heart's electrical conduction from the sinoatrial (SA) node to the atrioventricular (AV) node is interrupted.

Hemophilia: Occurs when blood has an inability to coagulate (form a clot) properly when needed. The patient is lacking an essential clotting factor.

Hypertension: High BP (greater than 140/90 mm Hg).

Ischemia: The temporary drop in blood flow to an organ or tissue.

Leukemia: Uncontrolled leukocyte production that invades blood cell–producing bone marrow. This is known as cancer of the blood.

Murmur: Sound resulting from blood flow turbulence through a narrowed or deformed valve.

Myocardial infarction (MI): Also called a heart attack. MI results from a lack of O_2, and some cardiac muscle necrosis occurs.

Phlebitis: A painful inflammation of a vein caused by venous infection, thrombosis, or intravenous fluid irritation.

Rheumatic heart disease: Damaged coronary valves resulting from rheumatic fever brought on by an untreated streptococcal upper respiratory infection.

Sickle cell anemia: Abnormal hemoglobin resulting in crescent-shaped RBCs that readily stick to capillary walls; hereditary. There are many signs and symptoms including anemia, pain crises, extremity numbness and swelling, fainting, and fatigue.

Tachycardia: A rapid cardiac rhythm greater than 100 beats per minute.

Thrombosis: A blood clot formation. A piece of the thrombus may break off and travel through the blood vessels; this is known as an **embolus.** The embolus may then become lodged in the lungs **(pulmonary embolism)** or in the brain, resulting in a stroke **(cerebrovascular accident [CVA])** or transient ischemic attack **(TIA).**

Varicose veins: Veins that have become distended and twisted. Most commonly, they are found in the superficial veins of the leg and are caused by long periods of standing over time, or they are seen as anal hemorrhoids.

Cardiovascular System Word Roots	
Root	Meaning
angi	Vessel
ather	Yellowish, fatty plaque
cardi, coron	Heart
isch	Deficiency, blockage
phleb, ven	Vein
sphygm	Pulse
ech	Sound

YOUR NOTES

_____

_____

_____

_____

_____

_____

Lymphatic and Immune System

Structures and Functions of the Lymphatic and Immune System	
Functions	**Cells, Tissues, Organs**
• Disease defense: active and passive immunity • Stores red blood cells • Returns excess interstitial fluid to blood • Produces lymphocytes • Transports lipids	• Lymph • Lymphocytes • Lymph nodes • Lymphatic vessels • Spleen • Tonsils: 3 pairs—palatine, pharyngeal, lingual • Thymus

Immunity

Immunity is the body's protection against infectious diseases and harmful organisms.

Active	Passive
Natural: Produced by body's production of antibodies after exposure to disease-causing organism	**Natural:** Maternal antibodies produced outside body and passed on while breastfeeding or in the uterus
Artificial: Acquired from immunizations composed of dead or weakened organisms, inactivated toxins, or recombinant DNA; body produces antibodies to become immune	**Artificial:** Acquired from immunizations composed of antibodies or globulins to fight specific disease-causing organisms readily, if exposed

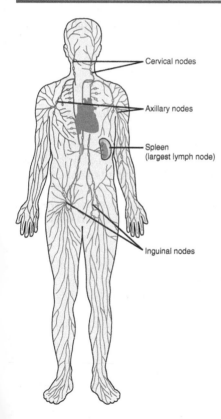

Lymphatic system.

Organization

Lymph

- Lymph is tissue fluid formed from plasma.
- It consists of water, electrolytes, metabolizing cell waste, and protein.

Lymphocytes

- Lymphocytes are WBCs formed in the red bone marrow.
- Lymphocytes mature within the spleen, liver, and lymph nodes to trap and destroy microorganisms and fight against pathogens. They are nongranular.
  - **T cells** mature in the thymus and reside in lymph tissue (spleen) and the blood.
  - **T cells** attack through cell-to-cell contact **phagocytosis (cell-mediated immunity).**
  - **B cells** mature in bone marrow and reside in lymph tissue (spleen) and the blood. B cells indirectly attack by secreting **antibodies (antibody-mediated immunity).**

Lymph Nodes

- Lymph nodes are pea-shaped clusters of lymph tissue that filter microorganisms from lymph as it flows through lymph vessels.
- Large cluster locations include **axillary lymph nodes, inguinal lymph nodes,** and **cervical lymph nodes.**

Lymphatic Vessels

- Lymphatic vessels form an extensive network, and every organ of the body has them.
- The lymph from the right arm and right side of head drains into the **right lymphatic duct.**
- Lymph from the rest of the body drains into the **thoracic duct.**

Spleen

- The spleen is the largest lymphoid organ.
- The spleen filters the blood and serves as a blood reservoir.

- This organ destroys old RBCs and has a role in erythropoiesis.

Tonsils

- There are 3 pairs of tonsils.
  - **Palatine:** Located at the opening of the oral cavity, this is the pair usually removed in a tonsillectomy.
  - **Pharyngeal (adenoids):** Also called adenoids, these are located near the opening of the nasal cavity in the upper pharynx. This pair is removed when they interfere with breathing.
  - **Lingual:** These are located in back of the tongue.

Thymus

- The thymus is mostly active in the development of the immune system during early life.
- It produces thymosin for maturation and the function of T-cell lymphocytes.

Diagnostic Testing and Procedures

Allergy testing: The methods used include the scratch test, patch test, intradermal test, and the radioallergosorbent test (RAST).

Complete blood count (CBC): This test profile includes a hemoglobin, hematocrit, RBC, and WBC count.

Enzyme-linked immunosorbent assay (ELISA): This screening test for HIV antibody presence is performed on venous blood and oral fluid samples. It is 85% accurate because of cross-activity from other viruses.

Liver function: This test measures the coagulation factors of prothrombin and fibrinogen.

WBC differential: This blood test determines the percentages of the different types of leukocytes present. The percentages change during infections, allergic responses, and certain diseases.

Western blot: This test is specific to individual viruses and is performed to confirm the diagnosis when a positive result from ELISA for HIV is found. It is more accurate than ELISA and may be performed on venous blood and oral fluid samples.

Common Diseases and Conditions

Allergies: Hypersensitivities result in inflammation, which may be delayed or immediate, to substances not usually recognized as foreign (contact dermatitis, anaphylaxis).

Autoimmune disorder: The immune system produces antibodies against its own cells (antigens). These disorders affect most body systems (rheumatoid arthritis, multiple sclerosis, Crohn disease, diabetes mellitus type 1, lupus, and more).

Immunodeficiency disease: Congenital or acquired; the immune system is incompetent or deficient, such as in the following disorders:

- **Severe combined immunodeficiency (SCID):** This is congenital. Children succumb to minor infections.
- **Acquired immunodeficiency syndrome (AIDS):** The most advanced stage of infection with the HIV virus is characterized by a significant decrease in immunity evidenced by a low T-cell count.

Systemic lupus erythematosus (SLE): This autoimmune disorder, also known as lupus, affects few or many organ systems. More female than male patients are affected. The actual cause is unknown, but SLE may result from drugs or bacterial infections. Some signs and symptoms include general body aches, weight loss (anorexia), "butterfly" rash on the face, sensitivity to sunlight, nosebleeds, and seizures.

Lymphoma: This general term describes benign or malignant tumors affecting lymphoid tissues. The 2 most common types are:

- **Hodgkin lymphoma (Hodgkin disease):** This malignancy with an enlarged spleen and lymphocytes known

as Reed-Sternberg cells generally occurs in young male patients.
- **Non-Hodgkin lymphoma:** This term describes all lymphomas other than Hodgkin lymphoma. It may be fast growing or slow growing. Malignancy is found throughout the lymph tissues. It generally occurs in older adults.

Mononucleosis (mono): This highly contagious viral infection is commonly known as "the kissing disease." Infection is from the Epstein-Barr virus or from cytomegalovirus (CMV). It is characterized by extreme fatigue, fever, sore throat, and an enlarged spleen and lymph tissue.

Splenomegaly: This term describes an enlarged spleen that is associated with an infectious disease.

Lymphatic and Immune System Word Roots	
Root	Meaning
lymph	Lymph
spleno	Spleen
thym	Thymus

YOUR NOTES

_____
_____
_____
_____
_____
_____
_____

Digestive System

Structures and Functions of the Digestive System

Functions	Cells, Tissues, Organs
• Digestion • Absorption • Elimination	• Mouth • Pharynx • Esophagus • Stomach • Small intestines and large intestines • Liver • Gallbladder • Pancreas

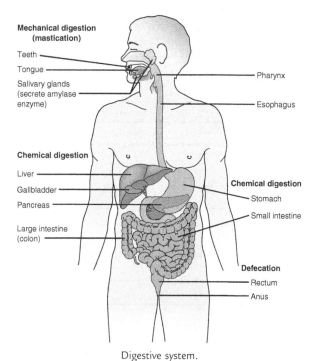

Digestive system.

Organization

The digestive tract consists of a series of chambers.

Mouth

- The oral cavity is where mechanical and chemical digestion starts.
- The act of **mastication** mixes food with saliva to form a **bolus.**
- The tongue has a **frenulum linguae,** tissue that anchors the tongue to the mouth floor.

Pharynx

- The pharynx is also called the throat.
- It passes the formed bolus to the esophagus.

Esophagus

- This is the "food tube" between the pharynx and the stomach.
- **Epiglottis:** This flap of tissue covers the larynx (windpipe) when swallowing so the bolus will enter the esophagus.
- **Peristalsis:** This involuntary rhythmic movement begins in the esophagus and moves first the bolus and then chyme through the digestive tract.

Stomach

- Consists of the following (beginning to end):
  - Esophageal sphincter: works to prevent food backing up into the esophagus
  - Fundus: upper portion of stomach
  - Body: middle portion of stomach
  - Pylorus: lower end of stomach
  - Pyloric sphincter: regulates rate at which partially digested food enters the duodenum
- Stomach wall is composed of **rugae folds** that allow the stomach to expand.
- The stomach mixes food with gastric acids and digestive enzymes to form **chyme.**

- It secretes gastric hormones and intrinsic factor (assists in absorption of vitamin B_{12}).

Small Intestine

- Most absorption of nutrients takes place here through the circular folds in the wall with finger-like projections called **villi.**
- This longest portion of the intestines is divided into 3 regions:
  - **Duodenum:** This is the 1st section of the small intestine (10 inches long). Bile from the gallbladder and pancreatic juices enter here; most digestion and absorption occur here.
  - **Jejunum:** This 2nd and middle portion (8 feet long) is the site of some digestion and absorption.
  - **Ileum:** The last part of the small intestine is 12 feet long.

Large Intestine

- The large intestine absorbs water and stores material until it is eliminated.
- No digestion takes place in the large intestine.
  - **Cecum:** This is a blind pouch where the ileum ends and the colon begins. The lower portion is the **appendix.**
  - **Colon:** Waste forms and moves through this organ by peristalsis. The colon has 4 parts:
    - **Ascending:** This is the 1st part of the colon and is located on the right side of the abdomen.
    - **Transverse:** This is the middle portion of the colon.
    - **Descending:** This is on the left side of the abdomen and leads to the sigmoid.
    - **Sigmoid:** This is S-shaped and connects the colon to the rectum.
- **Rectum:** This connects the sigmoid to the anus.
- **Anus:** This final portion of the digestive system is where feces are excreted.

Accessory Organs of Digestion

Liver: This organ produces bile and cholesterol. It stores glycogen and vitamins B_{12}, A, D, E, and K. The liver detoxifies blood and aids metabolism.

Gallbladder: This organ stores and secretes bile to aid in digestion, and it emulsifies fats.

Pancreas: As an **exocrine organ,** the pancreas produces pancreatic juices for digestion. It is also an **endocrine gland** that secretes insulin into the bloodstream.

Diagnostic Testing and Procedures

Colonoscopy, sigmoidoscopy, proctoscopy: These procedures are performed to view parts of the large intestine.

Lower gastrointestinal (GI) series: This procedure uses a barium enema to enhance x-rays of the lower GI tract.

Upper GI series: This procedure uses a barium swallow to enhance x-rays of the upper GI tract.

Ultrasonography: This procedure is used to produce an image of the gallbladder and bile ducts.

Common Diseases and Conditions

Anorexia: No appetite and an aversion to food, especially when the condition is caused by disease.

Anorexia nervosa: Voluntary starvation and excessive exercising. This false perception of body image and fear of gaining weight are characterized by being abnormally thin.

Appendicitis: Inflammation of the appendix possibly caused by blockage of it by feces, tumor, or infection. The **McBurney point** is the site of tenderness associated with appendicitis.

Botulism: Illness caused by toxins from *Clostridium botulinum*, usually acquired from ingesting contaminated food.

Cholelithiasis: Commonly referred to as a gallstone (calculus). A gallstone is a hard-mineral deposit formed in the gallbladder and bile ducts. Gallstones are known to be painful and to cause vomiting and mild jaundice.

Cirrhosis: The end stage of liver disease in which there is chronic liver cell destruction.

Colitis: Inflammation of the colon. This affects only the innermost lining, not the deep tissues.

Crohn disease: This chronic autoimmune inflammatory bowel disease is usually seen in the ileum. It penetrates every layer of tissue in the affected area.

Diverticula: Abnormal pouchings (pocketings) of organ walls, usually the colon.

Hemorrhoids: Dilated, inflamed, varicose veins of the rectum and anus.

Hepatitis: An inflammation of the liver. The 8 types are A, B, C, D, E, F, G, and H.

Hernia: A protrusion of an organ through the wall of the containing cavity.

Irritable bowel syndrome (IBS): Also known as "spastic colon." It is usually provoked by stress and/or gaseous foods and is characterized by bloating, constipation and/or diarrhea, cramping, and abdominal pain.

Ulcers: Lesions located in the mucous membrane lining of an organ.

Additional Information

Construction by adhesions: The abnormal growing together of 2 surfaces that normally would be separated.

Flatus: Gas in the digestive tract that is usually expelled through the anus.

Gavage: The process of feeding a person through a nasogastric tube.

Ascites: An abnormal collection of fluid in the peritoneal cavity.

Intussusception: One part of the small intestine slides into or over (telescopes) an adjacent part. It is sometimes found in infants and young children and is rare.

Vitamin K: Necessary for synthesis of prothrombin and several other clotting factors. Normal flora in the large intestine produces vitamin K.

Volvulus: A twisting or kinking of the intestine.

Digestion Word Roots	
Root	Meaning
an	Anus
cec	Cecum
cheil	Lip
chol	Gall, bile
cholangi	Bile duct
choledoch	Common bile duct
enter	Intestines, usually small
gastr	Stomach
gingiv	Gum
gloss, lingu	Tongue
hepat	Liver
lapar, celi	Abdomen; abdominal cavity
sial	Saliva
stomat, or	Mouth

YOUR NOTES

_____

_____

_____

_____

_____

_____

_____

Integumentary System

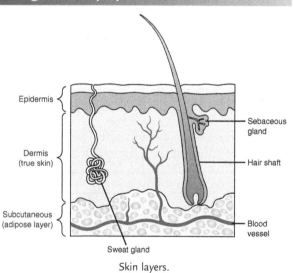

Skin layers.

Structures and Functions of the Integumentary System	
Functions	**Cells, Tissues, Organs**
• Controls body temperature • 1st line of defense from infection • Assists in preventing dehydration • Synthesizes and secretes vitamin D • Detects touch, pressure, pain, and temperature	• Skin: epidermis, dermis, subcutaneous • Sensory receptors • Glands: sweat, ceruminous, sebaceous **Accessory Components** • Hair • Nails

Organization

Skin

The skin is the largest organ; it covers all of the body.

- **Epidermis:** The outermost skin surface is made up of single cell layers (strata).
  - It contains **melanin** (the pigment that gives skin its color). Melanin is produced by melanocytes.
  - It prevents water loss from the body by way of **keratin.**
- **Dermis:** The "true skin," it is the middle layer containing the blood vessels, nerves, nerve endings, and glands.
- **Subcutaneous layer:** This is the innermost, fatty layer.
  - It contains adipose tissue and elastic fibers that adhere the dermis to muscle surfaces.
  - It provides the body with fuel, retains heat, and is a cushion for inner tissues.

Glands

The dermis layer contains the glands associated with the skin.

- **Sweat glands:** These produce and secrete sweat to assist in body temperature regulation and rid the body of waste.
- **Sebaceous glands:** These are located near hair follicles and secrete oily **sebum** to lubricate the skin and hair.

- **Ceruminous glands:** These are found in the ear and secrete **cerumen** (earwax) for protection.

Hair

- Hair is mostly composed of **keratin** tissue.
- It is found on most of the body's surface.
- The center of a hair shaft is called the **medulla**.

Nails

- Nails are composed of hardened **keratin (horny layer)** and are located on the tips of fingers and toes.

Diagnostic Testing and Procedures

Diascopy: This examination of skin lesions uses a flat glass plate held against the skin.

Lund-Browder Chart: This is a method to estimate the percentage of body that has been burned. It is more accurate than the "rule of 9" because it takes the patient's age and body proportions into consideration.

"Rule of 9": This is a quick method to estimate the percentage of body that has been burned. It is not accurate in children.

Surgical excision and biopsy: These procedures are performed for lesions, moles, and tissue for pathological study.

Sweat chloride test: This procedure detects cystic fibrosis (CF) by measuring the salt content of sweat.

Wood's light: This fluorescent light is used to diagnose particular skin conditions.

Common Diseases and Conditions

Acne: This is an inflammation of the sebaceous glands.

Albinism: This genetic condition is marked by the absence of melanin (pigment) in skin, hair, and eyes.

Alopecia: This term describes the absence or loss of hair to the entire body or body area.

Burns:

- 1st degree: A superficial burn involving just the epidermis, such as a rug burn. It results in very little edema.
- 2nd degree: A partial-thickness burn involving the epidermis and part of the dermis. Blistering and edema occur.
- 3rd degree: A full-thickness burn involving all 3 layers of skin, which has a pale or charred appearance with edema.
- If the body surface area affected is more than 15%, the burn is considered serious.

Carcinoma (skin cancer):

- Basal cell cancer: Located in the basal cell layer, this cancer is very slow spreading, and when diagnosed it is usually found on fair-skinned individuals.
- Squamous cell cancer: This involves the squamous cell layer and metastasizes more quickly than basal cell cancer.
- Malignant melanoma: Also known as melanoma. This most serious type of skin cancer occurs in the melanocytes. This usually begins with a change to a mole (size, shape, and irregular color and/or border) and metastasizes quickly.

Dermatitis: Inflammation of the skin causes itching and redness.

Diaphoresis: This term is used to describe excessive sweating.

Eczema: This continuous or returning form of dermatitis is possibly an abnormal reaction of the body's immune system. It causes itching, redness, cracking, oozing, blistering, or bleeding.

Furuncle: This is a boil.

Herpes: Painful blister-like sores are caused by a virus. Inadequate rest, poor nutrition, and stress may increase the likelihood of outbreaks.

% Total body surface area burn
Be clear and accurate, and do not include erythema
(Lund and Browder)

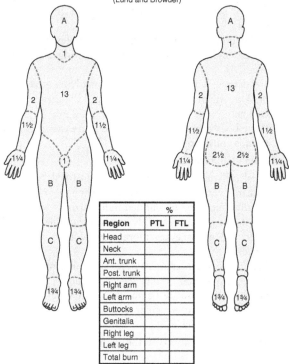

	%	
Region	**PTL**	**FTL**
Head		
Neck		
Ant. trunk		
Post. trunk		
Right arm		
Left arm		
Buttocks		
Genitalia		
Right leg		
Left leg		
Total burn		

Area	Age 0	1	5	10	15	Adult
A = ½ of head	9½	8½	6½	5½	4½	3½
B = ½ of one thigh	2¼	3¼	4	4½	4½	4¾
C = ½ of one lower leg	2½	2½	2¾	3	3¼	3½

Lund and Browder burn chart.

- Herpes simplex 1: Virus causing a cold sore or fever blister to lips, mouth, face; very contagious, spread through saliva
- Herpes simplex 2: Virus causing genital herpes; sexually transmitted

Herpes zoster: This acute viral infection is commonly known as **shingles**. The cause is the dormant varicella (chickenpox) virus reactivated later in life. It is characterized by painful skin eruptions that follow the route of inflamed nerves.

Impetigo: This is a very contagious bacterial skin infection caused by streptococcus or staphylococcus.

Keloid: This benign growth occurs in a scar or as a result of skin injury; excessive scar tissue is made up of collagen and fibrous tissues. The appearance of this scar is raised and often disfiguring.

Macule: This is a flat skin lesion that is white, brown, or red (freckle).

Nevus: This is a raised, congenital spot on the skin surface; a mole.

Papule: This term is used for a pimple.

Pediculosis: This condition is caused by an infestation by lice, usually on the head.

Psoriasis: This inflammation of the skin is evidenced by scaly red, raised patches on the skin surface covered with gray or silvery scales. Sometimes lesions form papules. It may be genetic or caused by environmental factors.

Scabies: This itchy skin condition is caused by a mite burrowing under skin.

Scleroderma: This condition causes the skin to thicken and become rigid.

Tinea: This fungal skin infection, also known as ringworm, can grow on skin, hair, and nails.

- Tinea capitis: Found on the scalps of children
- Tinea cruris: Found on the genital area (jock itch)
- Tinea pedis: Found between the toes (athlete's foot)

Urticaria: Commonly known as hives, this is usually seen as raised wheals caused by an allergic reaction or stress.

Vesicle: This is a fluid-filled, blister-like sac on the skin.

Integumentary Word Roots	
Root	**Meaning**
cutane, derm, dermat	Skin
hidr	Sweat
kerat	Horny tissue, hard
onych, ungu	Nail
trich	Hair
crypt	Hidden
heter	Other
myc	Fungus
pachy	Thick
rhytid	Wrinkles
xer	Dry

YOUR NOTES

Respiratory System

Structures and Functions of the Respiratory System

Functions	Cells, Tissues, Organs	
	Upper Tract	Lower Tract
• Inhalation: inhaling nutrients to body (e.g., O_2) • Exhalation: exhaling body waste products (CO_2) • Gas exchange: supplying and removing gases to and from blood • Maintains pH balance of the body • Produces sound • Traps and removes inhaled pathogens and debris	• Nose • Sinuses • Mouth • Pharynx • Epiglottis • Larynx	• Trachea • Bronchi • Alveoli • Lungs • Diaphragm • Pleura • Thorax

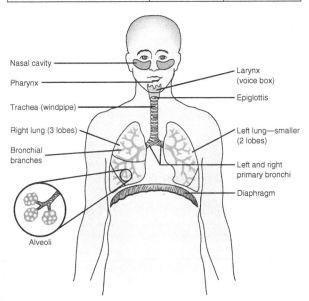

Nasal cavity

Pharynx

Trachea (windpipe)

Right lung (3 lobes)

Bronchial branches

Larynx (voice box)

Epiglottis

Left lung—smaller (2 lobes)

Left and right primary bronchi

Diaphragm

Alveoli

Respiratory system.

Organization

The upper respiratory tract, the trachea, and the bronchus comprise the passageway for air to the lungs. The exchange of O_2 and CO_2 takes place in the lungs.

Upper Respiratory Tract

- **Nose**
  - Lined with **cilia** and hair to clean air
  - Warms, cleans, and moisturizes air
- **Sinuses**
  - Air spaces in the bones of the face
  - Lined with **ciliated** mucous membrane
  - Warm, clean, and moisturize air
- **Mouth**
  - The mouth takes in extra air when needed, such as during exercise or when nasal passages are blocked.
  - The mouth does not have any moisturizing capacity. Inhaled air takes the available moisture, thus drying the mouth.
- **Pharynx (throat):** This serves as a passageway for air and food from the mouth to the **hyoid** bone.
- **Epiglottis**
  - Consists of a cartilage flap
  - Functions as a valve; moves to cover the larynx as you swallow

Lower Respiratory Tract

- **Larynx**
  - This contains the glottis and vocal cords (voice box) and is located just below the epiglottis.
  - It consists of cartilage and muscle.
  - It is a backup for the epiglottis. The epiglottis moves to cover the larynx, and then the muscles of the larynx squeeze shut.
- **Trachea (windpipe):** This tube is positioned anterior to the esophagus within the neck. Smooth muscle is reinforced with rings of cartilage; the rings are C-shaped

with the open end next to the esophagus. The rings prevent the trachea from collapsing.

- **Bronchi**
  - Two primary bronchi split off from the trachea, 1 to each lung.
  - Bronchioles split off as smaller branches from the bronchi.
- **Alveoli**
  - Air sacs at the bronchiole ends; 1 cell thick.
  - This is where exchange of gases occurs. O_2 enters surrounding blood capillaries and CO_2 enters alveoli from the surrounding blood capillaries. The process is known as **external respiration**.
- **Lungs**
  - The lung is the main respiratory organ.
  - In the thoracic cavity, the lung is protected by the surrounding bone structures (rib cage, sternum, vertebrae) and by the intercostal and diaphragm muscles.
  - The left lung has 2 lobes (the heart is also in the left thorax), and the right lung has 3 lobes.
- **Pleura:** The serous membrane lining the lungs has surfactant to lower the surface tension.
- **Thorax:** This cavity contains the lungs.
- **Diaphragm**
  - This domed muscle separates the thoracic and abdominal cavities.
  - On inhalation, the diaphragm contracts, creating room for inflation of lungs.
  - On exhalation, the diaphragm relaxes (assists lung compression).

Additional Information

Cilia: Tiny hair-like projections located on the surface lining of the trachea, bronchi, and just inside the nostrils. They function to filter incoming air and to move mucus or particles out of the respiratory tract. (Cilia are also located in other body systems.)

Expiratory reserve volume: The extra air forcibly exhaled after normal exhalation.

External respiration: The exchange of O_2 and CO_2 in the lungs and blood capillaries.

Functional residual volume: The amount of air left in the lungs after a normal expiration.

Inspiratory capacity (inspiratory reserve volume): The maximum amount of air inspired after normal expiration. This is measured by breathing in and out normally and then forcibly inhaling at the end of tidal volume.

Internal respiration: The exchange of O_2 and CO_2 between the capillaries and tissue cells.

Rales: The increased secretions in the bronchi causing crackling breath sounds.

Residual volume: The volume of air left in the lungs after forced expiration.

Tidal volume: The volume of air inspired and expired during a normal respiration.

Total lung capacity: The total volume of air that can be in the lungs at 1 time.

Vital capacity: The maximum amount of air expired after a maximum inspiration. It is not forced.

Wheeze: The squeaking, whistling breath sound caused by narrowed tracheobronchial airways. It occurs in asthma, bronchitis, and other respiratory disorders.

Diagnostic Testing and Procedures

Bronchoscopy: This procedure provides an interior view of bronchial air passages.

Chest x-ray: This is a radiological picture of the lungs.

Pulmonary function tests: This group of tests is used to measure various lung capacities such as the amount and rate of air taken in and released (spirometry).

Common Diseases and Conditions

Acute respiratory distress syndrome (ARDS) and **acute respiratory failure (ARF):** Sudden onset of lung dysfunction making breathing extremely difficult. It affects both lungs and is caused by trauma, sepsis, pneumonia, or shock.

Asthma: Affects bronchi and bronchioles. The airways become partially blocked by contraction of the muscle walls. The narrowed airways cause wheezing, chest tightness, or severe dyspnea; usually related to allergies, exercise, or environmental agents.

Atelectasis: Incomplete lung expansion. The absence of air in the lung(s) and alveoli causes structures to collapse. It may be caused by cancer, asthma, or pneumonia. Symptoms are dyspnea and hypoxia.

Bronchitis: An inflammation of the bronchi.

* **Acute:** Common complication of an ordinary cold, usually a secondary bacterial infection. Symptoms include fever, dyspnea, sneezing, yellow-green sputum, and productive cough.
* **Chronic:** One of the diseases of chronic obstructive pulmonary disease (COPD); leads to lung damage, eventual respiratory failure, and death. Symptoms are similar to those of acute bronchitis, but they occur over long periods and several times each year.

COPD: Various combinations of asthma, chronic bronchitis, and emphysema. COPD typically causes enlargement of the lung alveoli. This condition is usually progressive and obstructs the air exchange in the bronchi, alveoli, and lungs.

Croup: An acute virus affecting the larynx, trachea, and bronchi with inflammation and spasm. This disease of early childhood and infants causes a pronounced barking cough and hoarseness.

Cystic fibrosis (CF): Abnormally thick mucus secretions clogging the lungs and pancreas and resulting in impaired breathing. The cause is genetic.

Emphysema: Form of COPD in which enlargement and loss of alveoli and decreased elasticity of the lungs lead to a progressive loss of function. The usual cause is smoking or a previous history of smoking. The symptom is increasingly difficult, rapid, shallow breathing.

Pertussis (whooping cough): Contagious bacterial infection that causes inflammation in the upper respiratory system. This infection may be fatal to infants. A vaccine is available.

Pleurisy: Inflammation of the pleura that causes sharp pain with each breath taken. The cause may be injury beneath the pleura or influenza.

Pneumonia: Infection and inflammation of the lung tissue. Pus and other liquids present in the alveoli and bronchioles make it difficult for air to reach the alveoli. Causes may be bacteria, fungi, viruses, or inhaled agents. The type of pneumonia is named for the causative agent.

Pulmonary edema: Fluid accumulation in lungs from blood capillaries around alveoli resulting from a malfunction of the heart. It is associated with CHF. Symptoms are progressive dyspnea, nonproductive cough, and cyanosis.

Tuberculosis (TB): Infection with *Mycobacterium tuberculosis* causing nodules in lungs, damage to lung tissues, scarring where active bacteria are present, and dyspnea. TB will progress, if not treated, and be fatal. Symptoms include slight fever, fatigue, weight loss, unproductive cough, and eventual bloody, pus-filled phlegm.

Respiratory System Word Roots	
Root	Meaning
lob	Lobe
nas, rhin	Nose
pneum, pneumat, pneumon	Lung, air
pulmo	Lung

Respiratory System Word Roots—cont'd	
Root	**Meaning**
muc	Mucus
ox	Oxygen
py	Pus
spir	Breathe, breathing

YOUR NOTES

_____

_____

_____

_____

_____

_____

_____

Nervous System

Structures and Functions of the Nervous System	
Functions • Controls and integrates body activities • Adjusts body functions for homeostasis • Initiates thoughts and emotions • Generates sensations • Receptors for smell, taste, sound, and vision	**Cells, Tissues, Organs** **Central Nervous System** • Brain • Spinal cord **Peripheral Nervous System** • Spinal nerves and ganglia • Cranial nerves and ganglia

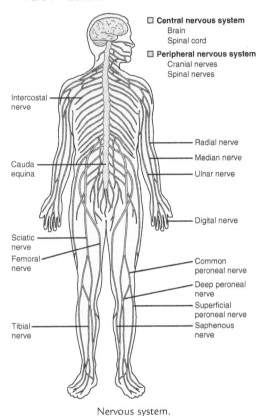

Nervous system.

Organization

Neuron

- The neuron is the **nerve cell** that carries nerve impulses to and from and within the CNS. These are the working cells of the nervous system.
  - **Cell body:** This holds the nucleus of the cell and other regular cell parts; however, it does not have a centriole

and therefore cannot reproduce. The cell body is protected in the brain, spinal cord, or ganglion.

- **Dendrite:** This extension of the cell receives and carries signals to the cell body.
- **Axon:** This cell part carries impulses from the cell body to other neurons or body tissues.
- **Myelin (lipid and protein) sheath**
  - Myelin covers the axon of a **PNS** cell. This is the **white matter** on nerve cells.
  - It is made from **Schwann cells;** gaps are called the **nodes of Ranvier.**
  - **CNS** neurons do not have a myelin sheath and therefore cannot be repaired. They are the **gray matter** cells (primarily cell bodies, interneurons, and unmyelinated fibers).
- **Synapse:** This gap between neurons and/or muscle tissue is designed so that impulses can travel in a single direction from axon to dendrite.
  - Released neurotransmitter chemicals assist or inhibit impulse transmission to cross the synapse to another cell.

Peripheral Nervous System (PNS)

The PNS consists of the nerves and ganglia located outside the CNS. A nerve consists of many neurons bundled together with blood vessels, wrapped in connective tissue. Types of nerves are as follows:

- **Sensory neurons:** These neurons transmit impulses from the rest of the body to the CNS.
- **Motor neurons:** These neurons transmit impulses from the CNS to muscles and glands.
- **Interneurons:** These CNS neurons are the bridge between sensory and motor neurons.

Somatic system: This system sends behavior information to and from the CNS to skeletal muscles.

- Afferent nerves bring sensory information from the different parts of the body (especially skin and muscles) to the CNS.

- Efferent nerves bring motor information from the CNS to the skeletal muscles.

Autonomic nervous system: This system sends behavior information from the CNS to smooth muscle, cardiac muscle, and glands.

- **Sympathetic nervous system:** Responsible for the automatic reactions to stress (the "flight or fight" response). For example, heart rate and strength increase, and bronchial tubes dilate.
- **Parasympathetic nervous system:** Responsible for the conservation or restoration of energy and elimination of waste. For example, heart rate decreases (with no direct effect on strength), and bronchial tubes constrict.

Cranial Nerves

I. Olfactory: Sense of smell

II. Optic: Vision

III. Oculomotor: Movement of eyeball and eyelid and regulation of pupil size

IV. Trochlear: Movement of eyeball

V. Trigeminal: Sensation in head and face; chewing

VI. Abducens: Eyeball movement

VII. Facial: Taste, facial expressions, and secretions of tears and saliva

VIII. Acoustic: Hearing and balance

IX. Glossopharyngeal: Taste, swallowing, and secretion of saliva

X. Vagus: Sensation in larynx, trachea, heart, stomach, and other organs; organ movement

XI. Spinal accessory: Movement of shoulders and head

XII. Hypoglossal: Tongue movement

Spinal Nerves

- Thirty-one pairs of spinal nerves extend from the spinal cord and are named for their originating vertebrae, as follows:
  - **Cervical plexus** (C1 to C4): These nerves supply the skin and muscles of the neck. The major nerve emerging from the plexus is the phrenic nerve (controls the diaphragm).

- **Brachial plexus** (C5 to C8, T1): These nerves supply the skin and muscles of the shoulder, arm, forearm, wrist, and hand.
- **Lumbosacral plexus** (T12, L1 to L5, S1 to end): These nerves supply the skin and muscles of the external genitalia, buttocks, lower abdominal wall, and lower extremities. The major nerve emerging from the plexus is the sciatic nerve (longest nerve in the body).

Central Nervous System

Brain

- The anatomical term for the brain is *encephalon*.
- The brain weighs 3 pounds.
- It is divided into 4 major areas: cerebrum, diencephalon, brainstem, and cerebellum.
- It is protected by the skull, meninges, and cerebrospinal fluid (CSF).
- **Main Sections of the Brain**
  - **Cerebrum** (left, right hemispheres)
    - This is the largest part of the brain.
    - It is the control center for sensory, motor, and intellectual function. It is covered with cerebral cortex of gray matter about 2 to 4 mm thick arranged in folds to fit as much of it into the space the skull allows.
    - The bulk of the cerebrum is composed of white matter.
    - It contains 10 to 14 billion neurons and synapses.
    - The 2 halves are not completely separate. The fissure between the hemispheres is bridged in the center by a band of white fibers called the **corpus callosum**, which serves to communicate between the left and right sides.
    - The left hemisphere is for logic, complex mathematics, and language. The right hemisphere is for creativity, music, and art appreciation.
    - Each hemisphere has 4 lobes: frontal, parietal, temporal, and occipital.
      - **Frontal:** This lobe controls speech and voluntary muscle movement.

- **Parietal:** This lobe processes sensory information from skin and controls depth perception, size, and shape.
- **Temporal:** This lobe controls the interpretation of sound and smell, the personality, behavior, emotion, and memory.
- **Occipital:** This lobe interprets visual information.

- **Diencephalon**
  - Comprising gray matter, the diencephalon contains the thalamus, hypothalamus, and pineal gland (these are briefly defined later under "Additional Information").
  - It is the link between where decisions are made and the body, which carries out those decisions.

- **Cerebellum**
  - The cerebellum is located below the cerebral hemisphere and attached to the posterior brainstem.
  - The cerebellum is known as the **little brain**.
  - It maintains muscle tone, balance, posture, and fine motor movement.

- **Brainstem (hindbrain):** This consists of 3 parts:
  - **Medulla oblongata:** The lowest part, it channels communication between the spinal cord and the brain.
  - **Pons (bridge):** This helps in regulating breathing.
  - **Midbrain:** This nerve tissue connects the pons to the lower part of the cerebrum. Vision and hearing reflexes are located here.

Spinal Cord

- The spinal cord is made up of gray and white matter. It serves as the pathway for impulses to travel to and from the brain.
- It begins at the **medulla oblongata** and extends to the 2nd lumbar vertebra in adults.
- The spinal cord is protected by the skull and vertebrae.
- It is enclosed in **meninges (membranes):** dura mater (outermost layer), arachnoid (lacy spiderweb), and pia mater (innermost layer).

CSF: This is made in the ventricles of the brain by masses of capillaries. The fluid is in the subarachnoid space, between the arachnoid and pia mater. CSF is clear, colorless, and watery. It functions to make the meninges into a fluid-filled cushion.

Additional Information

Blood-brain barrier: This mechanism of the capillary walls of the brain regulates what materials (e.g., drugs) in the bloodstream are permitted to enter the brain. Chemical excesses or deficiencies cause the arteries to either dilate or constrict until a balance is restored.

Hypothalamus: Located just below the thalamus. It regulates the emotional responses, body temperature, hunger sensations, thirst sensations, sleep-wakefulness cycles, pituitary and endocrine system action, and autonomic nervous system including heart rate, BP, respiratory rate, and digestive actions.

Pineal gland: Part of the endocrine system. It produces and secretes melatonin. This gland remains inactive during daylight but activates when darkness occurs. Melatonin helps control the sleep-wake cycle.

Plexuses (networks): Spinal nerve fibers converge to form these networks in the PNS.

Thalamus: Located below the cerebrum. It processes impulses relayed to and from the cerebrum and the sense organs.

Diagnostic Testing and Procedures

Cerebral angiography: This imaging procedure uses a contrast medium to view blood vessels of the brain.

Computed tomography (CT) scan: This imaging procedure uses a series of x-rays to create a cross-sectional, 3-dimensional picture of a bodily structure.

Electroencephalogram (EEG): This test measures the electrical activity of the brain.

Lumbar puncture: This procedure extracts CSF below L3 or L4 to obtain RBC and WBC counts.

Magnetic resonance imaging (MRI): Using a magnetic field and radio waves, this imaging procedure gives pictures of the brain's soft tissue.

Myelogram: This imaging procedure uses a radiopaque medium and x-rays to view the interior of the spinal cord.

Patellar, Babinski, Achilles, and corneal reflex tests: These tests are performed to evaluate motor neuron function.

X-rays (skull and spine): This radiograph imaging procedure is used to diagnose injuries, tumors, and spondylitis of the vertebrae.

Common Diseases and Conditions

Alzheimer disease (AD): Frontal and temporal lobe nerve cells die in this degenerative, dementia-like disease that impairs physical abilities, lessens intellect, and results in a gradual total memory loss.

Bell palsy: This infection causes 1-sided facial paralysis. It affects cranial nerve VII. It is usually caused by a herpes simplex reactivation and most often resolves in 2 weeks to 2 months.

Carpal tunnel syndrome: Pressure on the wrist median nerve causes pain and/or numbness, usually from repetitive motion over time.

Cerebral palsy: This brain damage occurs in utero or at birth and causes mental retardation, seizures, and spastic moves.

CVA (stroke): A sudden loss of neurological function caused by brain circulation block or vessel rupture. The loss of function depends on the location of the brain damage.

Epilepsy: A condition marked by periodic seizures caused by malfunction of the electrical activity of the brain.

Hydrocephalus: Excessive CSF in the brain causes elevated intracranial pressure and tissue death.

Meningitis: A viral or bacterial infection of the meninges covering the brain.

Multiple sclerosis: A progressive, debilitating disease caused by gaps in the white matter myelin sheath that produce increasing weakness, tremors, and vision problems.

Parkinson disease: A debilitating disease caused by an abnormally low supply of dopamine that produces an increase in body tremors, involuntary movement, and loss of balance.

Sciatica: Inflammation of the sciatic nerve. The symptom is sharp pain along the nerve and its branches, and this pain usually radiates from the buttocks into the hip and thigh areas.

TIA: A sudden loss of specific neurological function for which a full recovery within 24 hours is expected. A TIA serves as a warning of a possible upcoming stroke. It is caused by an embolus to the brain that is resolved by the body's circulatory system.

Seizure: A sudden surge of electrical brain activity commonly referred to as an "electrical storm." A seizure has an effect on behavior and on overall feeling for a short time. Various types of seizures have different effects.

- **Petit mal:** These seizures usually occur in childhood. The person has a mental shutdown ("goes blank") for up to 30 seconds. The patient does not know what is happening and after the episode does not know that it occurred.
- **Grand mal:** These may occur at any age. The patient falls down unconscious, goes rigid, twitches or jerks rhythmically, and then slowly regains consciousness. The episode is usually followed by deep sleep or confusion. The seizure may be preceded by an "aura" or warning.
- **Focal seizure:** These begin with uncontrollable twitching in a single part of the body (e.g., thumb) that spreads to surrounding structures and eventually the full body. The patient is conscious during this type of seizure.
- **Temporal lobe seizure:** An unconscious chewing motion may occur during this type of seizure.

Nervous System Word Roots	
Root	**Meaning**
cerebell	Cerebellum (hindbrain)
cerebr	Cerebrum
dur	Hard (dura mater)
encephal	Brain
radic, radicul, rhiz	Nerve root
esthesi	Sensation, sensitivity, feeling
phas	Speech
poli	Gray matter
psych, ment, phren	Mind

YOUR NOTES

Special Senses

Structures and Functions of the Special Senses	
Functions	Cells, Tissues, Organs
• Gustatory (taste)	• Papillae • Soft palate
• Olfactory (smell)	• Mucous lining (nasal epithelium)
• Vision	• Eyelids, eyelashes, eyebrows, tears • Lacrimal glands • Eyeball (3 layers and interior)
• Hearing • Sense of balance or position	• Outer ear • Middle ear • Inner ear

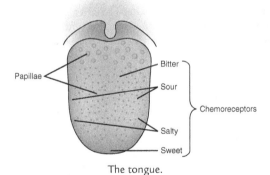

The tongue.

Organization

The senses function as a part of the nervous system. They have complex sensory organs unlike any other in the nervous system.

Gustatory Components

- Receptors for taste are mostly on the tongue and soft palate.
- **Papillae:** These are raised areas on the tongue that detect only 4 "tastes"—sweet, salt, sour, and bitter. Sensitivity to bitter-tasting substances is especially pronounced.

Olfactory Components

Smell receptors used in "tasting" and odor detection are located in the mucous lining of the upper part of the nose.

Vision Components

- Receptors for vision are in the retina.
- **Eyelids, eyelashes, eyebrows, and tears:** These protective structures clean and moisturize the eye.
- Lacrimal glands: These glands secrete tears and are located on the outside upper edge of each eye.

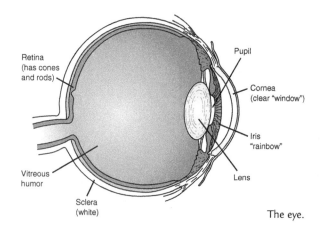

The eye.

- **Outer layer of eye**
  - **Sclera:** This is the "white of the eye."
  - **Cornea** ("window"): This transparent structure in the front of the eye helps focus light to enter.
- **Second layer of eye**
  - **Iris** ("rainbow"): This pigmented layer of muscles behind the cornea and in front of the lens enables more or less light to enter through an opening in the center known as the **pupil.**
- **Third layer of eye**
  - **Retina:** This lines the interior of the eyeball and is made up of **rods** (detects gray tones) and **cones** (light and color), with the greatest concentration at the back of the eye's interior.
- **Interior of eye**
  - **Lens:** Located behind the cornea and iris, the lens enables the eye to focus, a process called **accommodation** (see "Additional Information").
  - **Vitreous humor:** This jelly-like substance fills the chamber behind the lens. Its functions are to maintain the shape of the eye and to support the retina.

Hearing Components

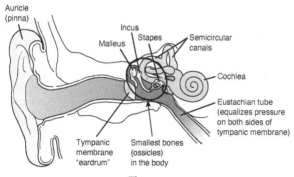

The ear.

- **Outer ear**
  - The external auditory canal extends from the pinna outward, inward, forward, and downward into the interior of the skull to the eardrum.
  - **Pinna (auricle):** This skin and cartilage make up the shape of the outside ear.
  - **Eardrum:** The auditory membrane vibrates as sound waves hit it.
- **Middle ear:** The tympanic cavity is connected to the nasopharynx via the **eustachian tube.**
  - **Malleus, incus, stapes (ossicles):** These bones move and pass vibrations from the middle to the inner ear.
- **Inner ear (labyrinth)**
  - **Vestibule:** This is a small chamber containing receptors for balance and position sense.
  - **Semicircular canals:** These canals also contain receptors for balance and position sense.
  - **Cochlea:** The stapes (middle ear ossicle) communicates with the cochlea. It is spiral shaped, contains fluid sacs and tubes, and has neural cells for hearing. Sound waves start fluid moving within the cochlea, so hairs bend to carry a nerve impulse to the acoustic nerve (cranial nerve VIII) and then to the temporal lobe to interpret sound.

Additional Information

Accommodation: This is the action of the eye lens to change its shape to bend light to focus it on the retina. This action allows the eye to adjust for differences in light because of distance; the lens becomes convex or concave. The greater the bulge, the more light will be bent.

Blind spot (optic disk): This is the region where the optic nerve leaves the eyeball and therefore does not contain rods and cones.

Eustachian tube (auditory tube): It begins in the middle ear cavity within the temporal bone. The area is full of air and is connected to the nasopharynx. The tube is normally flattened and closed, and it opens with yawning or swallowing. The tube's purpose is to equalize the pressure on both sides of the tympanic membrane.

Diagnostic Testing and Procedures

Audiometry: This test emits measured sounds to evaluate hearing.

Electrocochleography: This measures the electrical activity in the cochlea in response to sound to determine the cochlea's fluid pressure.

Refraction assessment: This procedure checks for necessary visual correction or glasses.

Tonometry: This is an intraocular pressure test to check for glaucoma.

Visual acuity test: The commonly known **Snellen eye chart** test is used to measure distance vision, near vision, and color vision by using the Ishihara methods for evaluation.

Common Diseases and Conditions

Amblyopia (lazy eye): This condition occurs when an eye is not used. It may be the result of misalignment by the muscles that control eye movement. The eye becomes progressively weaker, resulting in blurred vision, with the eye appearing to turn inward or outward.

Astigmatism: This uneven curvature of the cornea results in vision distortion.

Cataract: Cloudiness (opacity) of the eye lens results in vision degeneration, usually from aging.

Color blindness: The inability to distinguish certain colors, most commonly reds from greens, results from the absence or deficiency of a single type of cone. Red-green blindness is more common in both boys and men. It is usually present at birth and is inherited.

Conjunctivitis (pink eye): This allergic reaction or contagious bacterial or viral infection causes blood vessels in the conjunctiva to inflame, which turns the eye white to red or pink. Symptoms are red, itchy eyes, swollen eyelids, and a watery or sticky discharge.

Exophthalmia: Abnormal bulging (protrusion) of eyes out of their orbits is usually caused by hyperthyroidism.

Glaucoma: This is abnormally high pressure on the optic nerve. This condition can cause blindness because O_2 cannot reach the rods and cones.

Hypermetropia: Farsightedness results when the eye is too short from front to back. Light entering the eye is focused behind the retina.

Iritis: Inflammation of the iris tissue. Cells from the tissue may begin to flake off and float in the aqueous humor, which then interferes with vision. The affected eye becomes red and painful. If left untreated, iritis may cause acute glaucoma.

Macular degeneration: This progressive deterioration of the macula causes loss of central vision. It occurs because the retina no longer receives an adequate blood supply. This is the most common cause of vision loss in the United States.

Ménière disease: An increase of fluid in the semicircular canals of the ear results in symptoms of vertigo, nausea, progressive hearing loss, and tinnitus.

Myopia: Nearsightedness occurs when the eye globe is too long from the cornea to the retina, so that light entering the eye is focused in front of the retina.

Night blindness: This results from a lack of vitamin A.

Otitis externa: This inflammation or infection of the external ear canal is also known as **Swimmer's ear.** The most common cause is a bacterial infection.

Otitis media: This common middle ear infection in infants starts at the throat and travels up the eustachian tube; often the result of an upper respiratory infection.

Otosclerosis: Abnormal bone growth or immobilization of the stapes leads to conductive hearing loss. The cause may be genetic, and it is more common in both young and adult females.

Presbyopia: Hardening of the eye lens results in loss of lens flexibility, usually from aging. Seeing objects close up becomes more difficult.

Strabismus: This condition is commonly known as **cross-eyed** because of the poor alignment of eye muscles. Eyes do not focus together; one eye or both eyes will turn inward or outward. Common symptoms are blurred vision and poor depth perception.

Stye: An eyelash follicle infection causes a painful, red swelling that develops a white center and eventually bursts, thus relieving the pain.

Vertigo: This is the term for dizziness.

Special Senses Word Roots	
Root	Meaning
blephar	Eyelid
cor, core, pupil	Pupil
corne, kerat	Cornea
dacry, lacrim	Tear, tear duct
ocul, ophthalm	Eye
opt	Vision
cry	Cold
phot	Light
ton	Tension, pressure
acou, audi	Hearing
aur, ot	Ear
miring	Tympanic membrane (eardrum)
tympan	Eardrum, middle ear

YOUR NOTES

_____

_____

_____

_____

_____

_____

_____

Endocrine System

Structures and Functions of the Endocrine System

Functions	Cells, Tissues, Organs
• Secretes hormones; works with nervous system • Controls rate of certain chemical reactions • Helps transport substances through membranes affecting cell activities • Helps regulate water and electrolyte balance • Influences growth, development, and reproductive processes	• Hypothalamus gland • Pituitary gland (under brain) • Pineal gland (center of brain) • Thyroid gland (below larynx) • Parathyroid glands (thyroid lobes) • Adrenal glands (kidney tops) • Pancreas (in duodenum curve) • Gonads (sex glands)

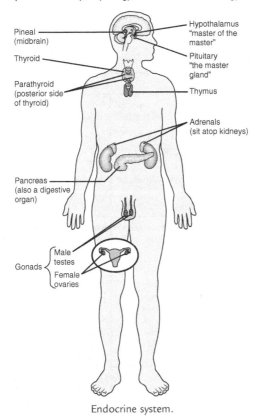

Endocrine system.

Organization

Hormone (by Gland)	Target	Major Functions
Anterior Pituitary		
Growth hormone (GH)	Bone, muscle, soft tissue	Stimulates tissue growth; decreases glucose
Prolactin	Mammary glands (breasts)	Initiates milk production; promotes milk gland production
Thyroid-stimulating hormone (TSH)	Thyroid gland	Growth, development, and thyroid activity as metabolism regulator
Adrenocorticotropic hormone (ACTH)	Adrenal glands (cortex)	Maintenance of gland, stimulates secretion of cortisol
Follicle-stimulating hormone (FSH)	Ovarian follicles, seminiferous tubules in testes	Women: stimulates development of ova and ovulation, secretion of estrogen Men: stimulates development and function of testes, production of sperm
Luteinizing hormone (LH)	Ovaries, testes—cells of Leydig	Development of corpus luteum, progesterone secretion; develops cells to make testosterone, stimulates secretion of testosterone
Posterior Pituitary		
Antidiuretic hormone (ADH, vasopressin)	Kidneys	Regulates water reabsorption within nephrons, determines urine concentration and volume
Oxytocin	Uterus, breasts	Stimulates birth contractions and causes milk ejection

Hormone (by Gland)	Target	Major Functions
Thyroid Gland		
Thyroxine (T_4)	Tissue cells	Increases metabolic rate
Triiodothyronine (T_3)	Tissue cells	Increases metabolic rate
Calcitonin	Bone	Inhibits bone loss; lowers blood calcium concentration
Parathyroid Glands		
Parathyroid hormone (parathormone)	Intestines, bones	Increases absorption of calcium into bloodstream; raises excretion of phosphates in urine
Adrenal Cortex (Outer)		
Cortisol (ACTH)	All cells except liver cells	Increases breakdown of proteins into amino acids; breakdown of fats; assists in stress; raises blood glucose
Aldosterone	Kidneys	Regulates blood pH; stimulates reabsorption of sodium in nephrons
Androgens	Gonads	Stimulates development of secondary sex characteristics (especially female)
Adrenal Medulla		
Epinephrine (adrenaline)	Smooth and cardiac muscle, blood vessels, liver cells	Raises heart rate, blood pressure, blood glucose levels

Continued

Organization—cont'd

Hormone (by Gland)	Target	Major Functions
Norepinephrine	Smooth, cardiac, and striated muscle	Constricts blood vessels, raises blood pressure; reinforces sympathetic nervous system
Pancreas Gland		
Glucagon	Liver cells, fat cells	Promotes release of glucose into blood
Insulin	All cells except brain cells	Promotes use and storage of glucose into cells
Pineal Gland		
Melatonin	Pituitary (LH), gonads	Regulates sexual development, timing of puberty
Thymus Gland		
Thymosin	Immune system	Stimulates T-cell production
Male Gonads (Testes)		
Testosterone	Sperm cells	Stimulates sperm production and secondary sex characteristics
Female Gonads (Ovaries)		
Estrogen	Breasts, uterus	Stimulates breast growth, uterus, and secondary sex characteristics
Progesterone	Uterine lining	Prepares uterus for pregnancy

Additional Information

Hypothalamus (master of the master gland): Regulates the pituitary gland; its secretions control the hormones secreted by the pituitary.

Metabolism: This is the sum total of all the chemical processes that take place in a living organism.

Pituitary gland: This is referred to as the **master gland.**

Steroid: These hormone-like substances either pharmaceutically produced or secreted by endocrine glands are used to relieve inflammation for conditions such as a strong allergic reaction, asthma, and other conditions.

Anabolic steroids: Male testosterone related, these substances are commonly used to increase muscle mass and strength. Mental side effects are violence, mood swings; physical side effects include breast development in male patients, testicular shrinkage, changes in body chemistry, and liver damage.

Syndrome: A set of symptoms that run (occur) together.

Diagnostic Testing and Procedures

Bone density x-ray: This is a radiographic image of the hip bone to measure the degree of calcium loss.

CT scan: This cross-sectional radiographic scan is performed to seek the cause of gland enlargement or the loss of hormone production.

Fasting plasma glucose test: This procedure determines a patient's normal blood glucose level.

Glucose tolerance test (GTT): A timed test to find the effective rate of glucose absorption into cells. It is usually performed during pregnancy to check for gestational diabetes.

Thyroid scan: This procedure is done by administering a pharmaceutical containing radioactive iodine. The scan rates a patient's thyroid activity for metabolic regulation and provides information about the size, shape, and location of any abnormalities.

24-hour urine collection: This tests for the concentration and levels of glucose, calcium, steroid, vitamin K, and other substances.

Common Diseases and Conditions

Acidosis: An abnormal accumulation of the acid products of metabolism. This is seen frequently in uncontrolled diabetes mellitus.

Acromegaly: A condition in which an abnormally high level of growth hormone is found in adults. The usual cause is a pituitary gland tumor.

Addison disease: This disease is caused by a slowly destroyed adrenal cortex and lowering of adrenocorticotropic hormone (ACTH), with resulting weight loss, nausea, abdominal pain, bronzed skin, and hypotension.

Cretinism: A congenital condition of hypothyroidism found in infants and children. It results in an abnormally developed brain.

Cushing syndrome: The symptoms caused by long-term exposure to high levels of ACTH or an adrenal-gland tumor. The evidence of this syndrome is a "moon face," thin limbs, and an obese torso.

Diabetes insipidus: In this disease, low levels of antidiuretic hormone (ADH) result in polydipsia, polyuria, dehydration, and dry skin.

Diabetes mellitus: A metabolic disorder caused by deficient insulin production in the pancreas or increased cell resistance to insulin.

- **Type 1:** Little or no insulin production, insulin-dependent diabetes mellitus (IDDM), onset before age 30 years, hereditary or resulting from a viral infection
- **Type 2:** Insulin resistance, non–insulin-dependent diabetes mellitus (NIDDM), adult onset; resulting from obesity or pregnancy; most common type

Goiter: A swollen neck from an enlarged thyroid is the result of an iodine deficiency or conditions that cause an underactive or overactive thyroid.

Graves disease: A form of hyperthyroidism (thyrotoxicosis) caused by destruction of the thyroid gland and evidenced by a high metabolic rate, exophthalmia, and anxiety.

Hashimoto disease: Chronic lymphocytic thyroiditis in which thyroid cells are destroyed by the body's own antibodies. This disease is autoimmune and is a condition of hypothyroidism.

Hyperthyroidism: Overproduction and secretion of thyroid hormones increase the metabolic rate and result in weight loss, sweating, and nervousness.

Hypothyroidism: An underactive thyroid causes a deficiency in hormone secretion, resulting in a decreased metabolic rate and in fatigue, depression, and cold sensitivity.

Myxedema: A severe type of hypothyroidism that is most common in women who are more than 50 years old. Causes may be obesity, thyroid removal, or radiation to the neck area. Some symptoms are as follows: fatigue; abnormally low body temperature; swelling of the face, hands, and feet; and hair loss.

Parathyroid tetany: Muscle spasms and convulsions resulting from hypoparathyroidism. This disorder results from low calcium levels in the body.

Seasonal affective disorder (SAD): This depressive mood disorder occurs during the winter months. It is possibly linked to increased melatonin production.

Endocrine System Word Roots	
Root	Meaning
acr	Extremities, height
calc	Calcium
dips	Thirst
kal	Potassium
toxic	Poison

YOUR NOTES

_____

_____

_____

_____

_____

_____

_____

Urinary System

Structures and Functions of the Urinary System	
Functions	Cells, Tissues, Organs
• Body waste elimination through blood filtration • Balance of fluids and electrolytes of body • Assistance in detoxification of liver • Regulation of blood chemical makeup	• Kidneys (2) • Ureters (2) • Bladder • Urethra

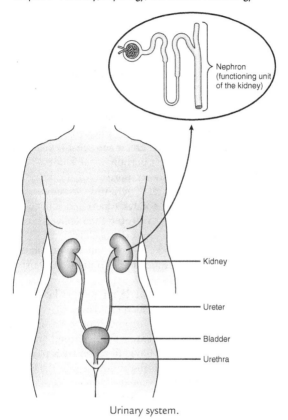

Urinary system.

Organization

Blood Circulation in the Kidney

- Blood enters the kidney through the renal artery, and waste products are removed as blood circulates through the nephrons within the kidney.
- Each minute the heart pumps about 1/5 (1,200 mL) of the body's blood supply through the kidneys.

Kidneys

This organ is 2nd to the brain in its complexity.

- The kidneys are located between the 12T and 3L vertebrae. They are behind the abdominal cavity.
- Kidneys secrete **erythropoietin,** which acts to stimulate the production of RBCs.
- Each kidney has a bean shape. The center of the kidney's concave side is called the **hilus.** The renal artery enters through the hilus, and the ureter and renal vein exit here.
- **Cortex:** This is the outer portion of the kidney.
- **Medulla:** This is the inner portion of the kidney and contains about 12 **renal pyramid** structures. Each pyramid connects with a **calyx** (duct) and joins a **renal pelvis** (urine reservoir). A **ureter** then collects the produced urine and delivers it to the bladder.
- **Nephrons:** These are the kidney's functioning units.
  - They carry out 3 functions: filtration, reabsorption, secretion.
  - There are approximately 1.25 million per kidney.
  - Each is surrounded by blood capillaries.
  - The anatomical features of a nephron are as follows:
    - **Glomerulus:** Blood enters the nephron here.
    - **Bowman's capsule:** Blood filtration takes place here.
    - **Proximal tubule:** Reabsorption begins; the concentration or chemical content of urine is determined.
    - **Loop of Henle:** Urine formation continues.
    - **Distal tubule:** The last area of urine formation.
    - **Collecting duct:** Urine formation is completed, and urine passes to the pyramids. Normally, glucose and amino acids are reabsorbed into the blood from the nephron tubules; however, if there are excess amounts in the blood, renal threshold occurs, and these substances become a part of the urine content.

Ureters

- The ureters are slender tubes that extend from the kidney's hilus to the lower surface of the bladder.

- Urine is propelled through the ureters by **peristalsis** and flows through a mucous flap into the bladder.

Bladder

- The bladder is a hollow organ that serves as the reservoir for urine.
- It has a mucous membrane lining of **rugae** cells that allow it to stretch to a 350- to 450-mL capacity. An empty bladder folds to become the approximate size of a walnut.
- An amount of 150 to 250 mL of urine is enough to stimulate **micturition** (voiding of urine).
- Urine exits the bladder via the **internal sphincter** (involuntary muscle), located where the urethra connects to the bladder.

Urethra

- The urethra conveys urine out of the body.
- It is about 4 cm long in a female body and 20 cm long in a male body.
- In a female body, the urethra leads directly from the bladder to the **urinary meatus.**
- In a male body, the urethra passes through the prostate before exiting through the urinary meatus.
- The urethra has an **external sphincter** (voluntary) that signals the urge to void.

Additional Information

Renal threshold: This refers to the occurrence of certain substances found in urine (glucose, amino acids) as a result of excessive amounts found in the blood. These substances are normally reabsorbed into the blood from the nephron tubules.

Urochrome: Pigment that gives urine its color. Color ranges from straw to amber yellow depending on liquid consumed, diseases, and medications.

Diagnostic Testing and Procedures

Dialysis: This is the artificial filtration of waste material from circulating blood.

Intravenous pyelogram (IVP): This x-ray procedure uses dye to evaluate the structure and function of the kidneys.

Routine urinalysis: Laboratory analysis of urine checks its physical properties, specific gravity, and basic chemistry.

Urine culture (UC): Performed to identify any pathogen(s) causing a problem. A clean-catch midstream specimen is required. A culture plate with an appropriate culture medium is incubated for 24 hours with the specimen on it. Bacteria that develop are identified and counted. Antibiotics are tested against the growing bacteria.

Urinary catheterization: This procedure removes or introduces fluids by inserting a sterile tube through the urethra and into the bladder.

24-hour urine collection: This procedure for urine collection allows testing of the urine sediment and content to diagnose various conditions.

Common Diseases and Conditions

Cystitis: Bladder inflammation resulting from a bacterial infection (usually *Escherichia coli*).

Glomerulonephritis: Inflammation of the glomeruli within the kidney nephrons affecting the filtration and reabsorption processes. With this condition the glomerulus loses the ability to be selectively permeable. Chronic glomerulonephritis is among the causes of chronic renal disease. It can occur as a complication of a streptococcal infection. It is caused by renal diseases, immune disorders, and bacterial infections. Some symptoms include drowsiness, coma, seizures, nausea, anemia, and high BP.

Hyperkalemia: An electrolyte-balance disorder caused by high potassium levels.

Polycystic kidney disease: A disease in which multiple cysts are produced in the kidney tubules and lead to kidney failure.

Pyelonephritis: A bacterial infection affecting the renal pelvis. An acute form usually results from a bladder infection moving up the ureters to the kidneys. The chronic form is caused by repeated undetected urinary tract infections (UTIs) that periodically affect the kidneys. Eventually the kidney becomes less efficient, and waste products accumulate in the body. Kidney or bladder stones can also be a source of infection. Symptoms include fatigue, frequent urination, itching skin, and nausea.

Renal calculi: Kidney stones of calcium that may block urinary flow. These stones are more common in men.

Renal failure: The gradual loss of renal function caused by repeated infections or by other diseases. It can be acute or chronic.

Urinary incontinence: The inability to maintain control of urination.

Wilms tumor: Forms on the outside of the kidney and metastasizes into the bloodstream, to the liver, and sometimes to the brain. It usually occurs in children less than 5 years old and has the highest survival rate of all childhood cancers. Symptoms may be weight loss, anorexia, vomiting, and blood in the urine.

Urinary System Word Roots	
Root	Meaning
azot	Urea, nitrogen
cyst, vesic	Bladder (vesic), sac (cyst [holding fluid])
hydr	Water
lith	Stone, calculus
meat	Meatus

Continued

Urinary System Word Roots—cont'd	
Root	**Meaning**
nephr, ren	Kidney
noct	Night
olig	Scant, few
pyel	Renal pelvis

YOUR NOTES

_____

_____

_____

_____

_____

_____

_____

Reproductive System

Structures and Functions of the Reproductive System	
Functions	**Cells, Tissues, Organs**
Female • Produce ova (singular, ovum) • Provide favorable environment for fetus to grow • Give birth to and feed newborn • Produce female hormones	Female • Ovaries • Fallopian tubes • Uterus • Vagina • Vulva • Breasts

Structures and Functions of the Reproductive System—cont'd	
Functions	**Cells, Tissues, Organs**
Male • Produce sperm • Deposit sperm into female reproductive system • Produce male hormone	Male • Scrotum and testes • Epididymis • Vas deferens • Seminal vesicles • Ejaculatory ducts and prostate gland • Cowper (bulbourethral) glands • Male urethra and penis

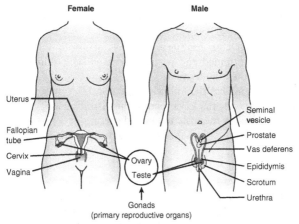

Reproductive system: (a) female; (b) male.

Organization: Female

Ovaries

These 2 glands manufacture ova and also secrete estrogen and progesterone.

Fallopian Tubes

- The tubes curl around the top of each ovary and connect to the top corners of the uterus to transport ova to the uterus.
- Fertilization by sperm occurs here.

Uterus

- The uterus is a hollow, muscular organ that contains and nourishes the developing embryo and fetus.
- The top of the uterus is called the **fundus.**
- The upper 2/3 is called the **uterus,** and the lower 1/3 is called the **cervix.**
- The inner wall of the uterus is called the **endometrium.**

Vagina

- The vagina is a muscular tube that leads from the uterus to outside the body.
- The inner layer has rugae cells for expansion.
- It is surrounded and partially covered by a thin membrane called the **hymen.**
- The vagina has the following functions:
  - It serves as the lower end of the birth canal.
  - It receives the male organ and sperm.
  - It provides a passageway to the outside for menstrual flow.

Vulva

- The vulva is a collective term for the external genitals.
  - **Mons pubis:** The fatty tissue over the pubic bone.
  - **Labia majora (vulval lips):** The 2 folds of skin tissue that enclose and protect the urethral and vaginal openings. There is hair on the outside.
  - **Labia minora:** A modified form of folded skin tissue, similar to the labia majora. These folds provide further padding and protection to the area.
  - **Clitoris:** Erectile tissue that is similar to a penis. It is covered by a **prepuce.**

- **Skene (urethral) and Bartholin (vaginal) glands:** They secrete mucus and lubricating fluid.

Breasts

- Breasts are the mammary glands that produce milk.

Organization: Male

Scrotum and Testes

- The testes are suspended in a sac of loose skin (scrotum).
- Before birth, the testes move from the abdominal cavity to the scrotum.
- The testes produce sperm.

Epididymis

- This tightly coiled tube is attached to the side of each testis.
- Sperm mature and are stored here.
- One end is connected to the testes; the other end leads into the vas deferens.

Vas Deferens

- These tubes move the sperm from the epididymis to the seminal vesicles.

Seminal Vesicles

- Glands that secrete a fructose-rich fluid. This fluid mixes with sperm passing through the vas deferens.

Ejaculatory Ducts and Prostate Gland

- **Ejaculatory ducts:** The merging of the vas deferens and seminal vesicles. The ducts pass through the middle of the prostate "donut hole" and join the urethra.
- **Prostate gland:** Has a donut-like shape that encircles the ejaculatory ducts. The prostate gland secretes a thin alkaline fluid that is added to the semen. It makes up 60% of the semen.
  - The fluid protects sperm from acids as it passes through the urethra.

Cowper or Bulbourethral Glands

- These glands secrete an alkaline fluid that makes up 5% of semen.

Urethra and Penis

- **Urethra:** A 20-cm-long tube that extends from the ejaculatory ducts to the tip of the penis
- **Penis:** The organ for copulation and urination
  - It contains erectile tissue that becomes engorged with blood, which stiffens the penis when stimulated.
  - The erection enables entry into the female vagina, where sperm is ejaculated.
  - The penis **glans** is the penis tip and is slightly wider than the rest of the organ.
  - The **prepuce** (foreskin) extends over the glans.

Additional Information

Apgar scoring system: The initial tests to assess the health of a newborn immediately after birth. Five signs are checked and scored: heart rate, respiratory rate, muscle tone, reflex irritability, and color.

Braxton-Hicks contractions: Uncoordinated and irregular contractions of the uterine muscle. These contractions occur frequently in the last month and sometimes earlier in pregnancy before labor.

Chadwick sign: A thickening of the vagina and the development of a purplish color in both the vagina and cervix.

Embryo: The term for a fertilized egg through 8 weeks of development.

Fimbriae: Finger-like projections on fallopian tubes that produce a pulling action on an ovum to draw it into the tubes after rupturing from the ovary.

Gestation: The period of pregnancy from fertilization to birth.

Goodell sign: The softening of the cervix 5 to 6 weeks after fertilization.

Menarche: The initial onset of female menses. It usually occurs between 9 and 15 years of age.

Menopause: The cessation of menstruation. It usually occurs around 48 to 50 years of age.

Menstruation (menses): The shedding of the endometrial lining because of nonpregnancy. It occurs approximately every 28 days.

Mitosis: This is the process describing 1 cell beginning to multiply through division.

Naegele rule: A formula to calculate the estimated date of confinement (EDC) or estimated date of delivery (EDD).

Parturition: The process of labor and delivery.

Perineum: An area of muscle located between the anus and the external genitals. It provides support for internal organs of the pelvic cavity.

Placenta: This spongy structure forms on the uterine wall during pregnancy and is joined to the fetus by the umbilical cord. It permits exchange of wastes, nutrients, and O_2 between the maternal and fetal systems. It is also a temporary endocrine gland and secretes human chorionic gonadotropin early in pregnancy as it develops.

Quickening: A pregnant person's initial awareness of the movement of the fetus within the uterus. It usually occurs between 18 and 20 weeks of gestation.

Teratogen (potent): The term used to describe toxic substances (alcohol, various drugs, various pathogens) that are able to cross the placental membrane and harm the developing embryo. The term means "monster producing."

Zygote: The fertilized egg cell produced when the sperm head unites with the nucleus of the ovum.

Diagnostic Testing and Procedures

Female Patients

Amniocentesis: This procedure uses a needle inserted into the amniotic sac to remove fluid for analysis.

Cesarean section: This is the surgical removal of a fetus from the mother. It is performed when the delivery process is difficult or hazardous and poses high risks for the pregnant person and/or fetus.

Colposcopy: The visual examination through a colposcope of the vaginal wall and cervix for any abnormal cells.

Dilation and curettage (D & C): This procedure dilates the cervix and scrapes the walls of the uterus to remove tissue.

Episiotomy: Clean surgical cut in the perineum done during labor. This area of muscle is under a great deal of stress during childbirth. The procedure is performed to prevent irregular and deep tearing.

Hysterectomy: Surgical removal of the uterus. The fallopian tubes and ovaries may be removed at the same time, for various reasons.

Mammogram: This is an x-ray of the breasts.

Pap smear (Papanicolaou test): This procedure takes a cell scraping of the cervix and vagina to test for abnormal cell growth.

Tubal ligation: A sterilization procedure accomplished by severing, knotting, or blocking the fallopian tubes.

Male Patients

Circumcision: The surgical removal of the foreskin (prepuce) of the penis.

Prostate-specific antigen (PSA) test: This measures the blood level of the PSA protein released by the prostate. It is used as an indicator for prostate cancer.

Vasectomy: The removal or knotting of the vas deferens for sterilization.

Common Diseases and Conditions

Female Patients

Cystocele: The outpouching of the bladder. It protrudes into the vagina and may cause urinary urgency.

Eclampsia (toxemia of pregnancy): This condition causes elevated BP, edema, and protein in the urine. If left untreated, it causes death.

Ectopic pregnancy (extrauterine): This condition requires surgery because the fetus has implanted outside the uterus.

Endometriosis: The presence of endometrial tissue outside the uterus. The condition is known to cause pain, cysts, and tumors.

Pelvic inflammatory disease (PID): A widespread bacterial infection of the reproductive organs.

Placenta previa: A placenta that is attached to the lower uterine wall and partially or fully blocks the birth canal.

Premenstrual syndrome (PMS): This is characterized by symptoms of anxiety, bloating, irritability, headache, and depression.

Infants

Down syndrome: This includes mild to severe mental retardation of an individual born with an extra chromosome (usually number 21).

Fetal alcohol syndrome: Birth defects such as facial deformities and mental and neurological development damage are caused by alcohol consumption during the embryonic period of pregnancy.

Phenylketonuria (PKU): Excess accumulation of phenylalanine occurs when a defective enzyme cannot metabolize the substance. It can cause brain damage.

Sudden infant death syndrome (SIDS): This occurs when the autonomic respiratory system stops.

Spina bifida: This birth defect exposes the spinal column, usually in the lumbar region.

Male Patients

Benign prostatic hypertrophy: An enlargement of the prostate that is commonly seen in men more than 50 years old.

Cryptorchidism: The failure of the testes to descend into the scrotum before birth.

Epididymitis: Inflammation of the epididymis causing pain on urination as well as pain and swelling of the scrotum.

Hydrocele: An accumulation of fluid within the testes.

Sexually Transmitted Diseases

AIDS: The advanced stage of infection with the HIV virus characterized by a significant decrease in immunity. At this time, a cure does not exist.

Chlamydia: A genitourinary infection caused by *Chlamydia trachomatis*. This is the most common sexually transmitted disease. It can cause a female patient to develop PID.

Condyloma: Wart growths located on the external genitalia are known to cause cervical cancer.

Gonorrhea: This genital mucous membrane inflammation is produced from exposure to *Neisseria gonorrhoeae*.

Herpes genitalis: A viral infection consisting of painful fluid-filled vesicles on the genitals. It can cause female cervical cancer.

Syphilis: A multistage genitourinary infection by *Treponema pallidum*. It is characterized during the disease's 1st stage by the lesions (chancres) on any organ or body part.

Trichomoniasis: A genitourinary parasitic *(Trichomonas vaginalis)* infection that can result in vaginitis.

Reproductive System Word Roots	
Root	Meaning
arche	1st, beginning
colp, vagin	Vagina
culd	Cul-de-sac
episi, vulv	Vulva

Reproductive System Word Roots—cont'd	
Root	Meaning
gynec, gyn	Woman
hyster, metr, uter	Uterus
mamm, mast	Breast
men	Menstruation
oophor	Ovary
salping	Fallopian tube
andr	Male
balan	Glans penis
epididym	Epididymis
orchid, orch, test	Testis
vas	Vessel, duct

YOUR NOTES

_____

_____

_____

_____

_____

_____

_____

Sample Certification Test Questions

Now that you have studied this chapter, here are some sample certification test questions for you.

1. The transparent anterior part of the sclera is the

   A. Iris
   B. Pupil
   C. Retina
   D. Cornea
   E. Pinna

2. The definition of cilia is

   A. Mucus-secreting cells in the lower bronchial tree
   B. Structures in the airways that trap and hold foreign material
   C. Tiny hair-like structures in the airways that sweep mucus up and out of the lungs
   D. Cells composed of macrophages that destroy inhaled pathogens
   E. Collecting ducts joining the renal pelvis located within kidneys

3. The diagnostic term myopia is defined as

   A. Double vision
   B. Condition of the white pupil
   C. Pain in the eye
   D. Farsightedness
   E. Nearsightedness

See the Appendix for the answers.

Remember to use Edge after you finish this chapter to test your knowledge. Directions for how to access Edge, as well as your access code, are located on the inside front cover of this text.

Chapter 4

Psychology and Interpersonal Communication

The importance of psychology and interpersonal communication to the profession of medical assisting cannot be emphasized enough. Each area is a fundamental part of all the roles of a medical assistant. Your understanding of these areas affects your contact with fellow coworkers, patients, physicians, and others in the workplace setting. The chapter begins with an overview of 3 influential ideas in psychology, followed by forms of listening. The chapter concludes with nonverbal communication, barriers to therapeutic communication, defense mechanisms, and finally psychological disorders.

Information regarding psychology and interpersonal communication content within the various national certifying exams may be found in Chapter 1.

Remember to use Edge after you finish this chapter to test your knowledge. Directions for how to access Edge, as well as your access code, are located on the inside front cover of this text.

Psychological Theories

The theories of psychology provide a basic understanding of human emotion and behaviors that are helpful to a medical assistant and other health-care workers. Later in this chapter, emotional and behavioral problems that make therapeutic communication difficult are presented to gain insight into human behavior and illness.

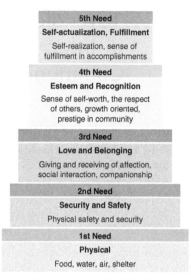

Maslow's hierarchy of needs.

Abraham Maslow proposed that people have categories of needs and these needs are arranged in a hierarchy. Maslow believed the following:

- People are motivated to satisfy or maintain the conditions that will first meet their lower-level needs.
- Generally, a person does not progress to the next level until the needs of the previous level have been met.
- People are protective of themselves, and any action that stands in the way of their basic needs, or endangers the defenses that protect them, is considered a threat. A person may respond negatively, even violently, to such a threat.

Erikson's Life Span Development

Erik Erikson developed 8 stages of physical, psychological, and emotional growth in humans based on age. By understanding the growth stages, medical assistants and other health-care workers will enhance their communication skills with patients in such areas as patient education.

Life Span Development	
Age (years)	The Expected Development
Infant: 0–1 *Trust vs. Mistrust*	The beginnings of familiarity and trust of surroundings, persons, and the future
Toddler: 2–3 *Autonomy vs. Shame and Doubt*	Exploring environments, developing self-control and control of environment
Young child: 3–6 *Initiative vs. Guilt*	Curiosity, learning new things, thinking creatively, beginnings of moral judgment and becoming purposeful
School-age child: 7–12 *Industry vs. Inferiority*	Exposure to people outside of family; learning through success and failure experiences in education, sports, and social settings
Adolescent: 12–18 *Ego Identity vs. Role Confusion*	Finding one's place in society; personal identification development
Young adult: early 20s *Intimacy vs. Isolation*	Beginnings of responsibilities in career, family, marriage; ability to love and commit; the young adult may change familiar group settings
Middle adult: late 20s–50s *Growth vs. Stagnation*	Teaching, writing, raising a family, and social activism; fulfilling life goals
Old adult: 60s *Integrity vs. Despair*	Reflecting on one's life concerning usefulness, fulfillment, physical health, and death

Elisabeth Kübler-Ross' "Stages" of Death and Dying

The medical assistant's role is to see the level of need being threatened. Nothing threatens the feeling of safety and security more than an illness, particularly in a dying patient experiencing stress and anxiety related to the dying process.

"Stages" of Death and Dying	
1st: Denial	A buffer against the harsh reality by denying existence of the problem: "No, not me."
2nd: Anger	Rage at the unfairness of the situation: "Why me?"
3rd: Bargaining	Spiritual bargaining with God and/or health-care workers: "I'll be good if I can have 1 more day."
4th: Depression	2 parts: 1. Quiet grieving, severe sadness 2. Realizing the loss of self, job, family
5th: Acceptance	Resigned to fate and planning for it, possibly with a sense of calm and peacefulness; fear of dying is eliminated

- The stages are not always distinct from each other; they may overlap.
- A person may repeat or skip stages.
- These stages enable us to understand all grieving people, who are facing death, loss of a loved one, amputation, loss of various body functions, loss of a preferred life-style, economic loss, or divorce.

Forms of Listening

Active Listening

Active listening involves showing awareness of what is being communicated and providing feedback; it is a 2-way interchange. The 5 techniques for active listening are as follows:

- Giving your full attention
- Nodding
- Smiling
- Asking questions
- Taking notes

Evaluative Listening

Evaluative listening is giving your full attention to the message transmitted to ask the most appropriate question(s) for clarification and understanding.

- This provides an immediate response and opinion.
- It is especially important in telephone communication.
- It avoids selective hearing.

Passive Listening

- No feedback is required.
- The listener is an audience member.

Nonverbal Communication

Communication is the sharing of information. It is how we interact with and relate to one another. Interactions require us to react or respond to others and observe how they react and respond to us. We begin to learn communication as infants. Some forms are automatic, but most communication is learned as the result of interactions with others.

- Nonverbal communication, or **body language,** is the expression of a person's attitude transmitted by posture, facial expression, touch, eye contact, or the spatial relationship between communicating parties.
- Your self-concept determines your behavior: how you react to the world in general and those around you. Most

of your communication is decided by the desire to preserve and increase your self-image. How you choose to communicate determines your relationships with those around you.

- Your attitude affects all communication you have with others. Attitude is 90% of who you are to others and what you represent to them. The following are examples: "She's got a bad attitude" (someone who expresses negative emotions) or "She gives off good vibes" (someone who makes you feel good and comfortable).
- Recognizing human behaviors and communicating effectively are essential to success in the field.

Proximity

- Proximity refers to the distance you are from the personal space area that surrounds someone.
- Observing space boundaries (comfort zone) between patient and caregiver shows respect for the patient.
- Culture, age, and gender can influence a patient's sense of personal space.
- "Personal space": 1.4 to 4 feet
- "Social space": 4 to 12 feet
- "Public space": 12 to 25 feet

Touch

- Touch is a powerful form of nonverbal communication.
- In a medical setting, a touch to the shoulder, forearm, or hand can show sensitivity and concern if it is used on someone who welcomes it.
- Touch can be seen as an invasion of privacy.
- Culture, age, gender, and family history influence a patient's understanding of touch.

Kinesics

Kinesics is the study of body movements and gestures as a form of nonverbal communication.

Kinesics	
Behavior	May Indicate
Tapping foot	Restlessness
Drumming fingers	Indifference, apathy
Head scratching	Uncertainty, bewilderment
Eye contact	Looking away or down: noninterest, avoidance, or respect (culture is a factor) Looking directly: interest
Gesturing with hand or arm movements	Emphasis of ideas and emotions, need to enhance message
Leaning forward toward a person	Interest
Posture	Standing or sitting erect: self-confidence Slumped posture: sadness or lack of confidence

Communication Terms

Accountability: To be responsible for actions and words

Empathy: Putting oneself in another person's place to realize that person's feelings

Nonjudgmental: To be fair or unbiased when communicating with others, as should be evident in facial expression, body language, and responses made

Nonlanguage: Sounds made while the message is transmitted, such as crying, laughing, humming, grunting, and sighing

Paralanguage: The way a message is transmitted, rather than the words used: the volume, pitch, voice tone, pronunciation, speed, and sentence structure

Perception: Being aware of your own feelings and the feelings of others

Communication Barriers

Behavior and Conditions

Giving unwanted advice: Most people do not like being told what they should or should not do. As a medical assistant, it is outside your scope of practice to offer advice to patients.

Using medical terminology: Medical terms and abbreviations should not be used unless they are explained.

Manipulation: Influencing or controlling artfully or deceptively because of the need to be in control. The individual cannot tolerate a dependent role. Manipulative patients may cancel appointments or not show up, or they may change their prescribed treatments.

Prejudice: Having a negative opinion or bias toward an individual.

Stereotyping: Believing that all group members (e.g., race, religion) share the same attitudes, attributes, or appearances.

Negative body language: This includes facial frowning, lack of eye contact, folded arms or crossed legs, and poor voice tone.

Disorientation: Loss of memory for time, person, and place is a communication barrier.

Introjection: A person identifies with the attitudes or characteristics of another individual.

Noise: Interruptions and noise (within the room or just outside) interfere with communication.

Defense Mechanisms

Fear, insecurity, or not knowing what else to do may keep you or a patient from communicating in a positive way. People use the following behaviors as techniques for dealing with uneasy situations they encounter in daily living.

Denial: Someone fails to recognize or acknowledge the existence of anxiety-provoking information.

Displacement: Emotional impulses are redirected toward a substitute person or object that is less threatening or dangerous.

Inversion: The patient does the opposite of what he or she wants; he or she reverses feelings about someone after being rejected by that person. For example, an individual may be rejected by someone he or she loves and then conclude it is best to hate that person to deal with the rejection.

Projection: One's own unacceptable urges or qualities are attributed to others.

Rationalization: One's actions or feelings are justified with socially acceptable explanations instead of one's true motives or desires.

Reaction formation: Someone thinks or behaves in extreme opposite of the unacceptable urges or impulses.

Regression: A person retreats to behavior characteristics of an earlier stage of development (e.g., sucking a thumb).

Repression: Anxiety-producing thoughts, feelings, or impulses are completely excluded from consciousness. Repression is a basic defense mechanism.

Sublimation: This is a form of displacement. For example, an unwanted sexual urge may be rechanneled into productive nonsexual activities.

Suppression: An unpleasant past is deliberately put aside or forgotten. This is the conscious form of repression.

Psychological Disorders

Psychological disorders are abnormal behavior patterns that affect one's ability to function or that cause psychological discomfort. Common disorders include the following:

Anxiety: Abnormally high tension, worry, or apprehension that interferes with daily activities and relationships; can be moderate to severe

Anorexia nervosa: A disorder in which calorie intake is severely restricted because of a heightened fear of weight gain

Bipolar disorder (manic depression): The occurrence of extreme mood swings, highs and lows, that affect someone's ability to function

Bulimia nervosa: A disorder identified by repeated episodes of binge eating followed by purging

Dysphoria: Depression and unrest without an apparent cause

Hypochondriasis: The belief that one has a disease despite reassurances that the disease is not present

Major depression: Profound loss of all hope, feelings of sadness, low self-esteem, and loneliness affecting the body and mind and causing physical and mental problems

Seasonal affective disorder (SAD): Depression that occurs mostly in the fall and winter

Obsessive-compulsive disorder: Behavior involving repetitive thoughts and actions

Panic attack: Sudden extreme anxiety resulting in sweating and rapid heartbeat and breathing

Paranoia: A show of persistent persecutory delusions or delusional jealousy, possibly with schizophrenic symptoms

Phobia: An extreme or irrational fear of a thing, environment, or situation

- **Agoraphobia:** Fear of being in public places outside of home
- **Acrophobia:** Fear of high places
- **Claustrophobia:** Fear of being confined in any space
- **Hydrophobia:** Fear of water
- **Social anxiety disorder:** Fear of being judged or criticized while performing routine behaviors in front of others at social gatherings

Post-traumatic stress disorder (PTSD): A response to physical or psychological trauma, usually long lasting, with symptoms that can include recurring flashbacks, nightmares, sleeplessness, loss of interest in things previously cared about, anger, irritability, and feeling emotionally cut off

Schizophrenia: A psychosis evidenced by delusions, hallucinations, and disorganized speech and behavior

Somatization: Recurrent and multiple body (any organ system) complaints with no physical basis

Other Illnesses

Autism: Characterized by severely impaired social or communications skills, often with repetitive or primitive behaviors, and a preoccupation with inner thoughts

Confabulation: A behavioral reaction to memory loss in which a patient fabricates ideas and uses inappropriate words to fill in forgotten information; seen in dementia and other conditions such as stroke

Dementia: A disease syndrome, also known as chronic organic brain syndrome, exhibited by a loss of recent memory and progressing to loss of orientation (time, person, place), with mental deterioration resulting from brain disease

Tourette syndrome: Uncontrollable motor tics, facial tics, verbal grunts, and use of profanity

---

YOUR NOTES

_____

_____

_____

_____

_____

_____

_____

Sample Certification Test Questions

Now that you have studied this chapter, here are some sample certification test questions for you.

1. Which of the following does Maslow consider a 3rd-level need?

- A. Shelter
- B. Belonging
- C. Safety
- D. Respect
- E. Esteem

2. Nonverbal communication is the language

- A. We learn as infants
- B. We learn as toddlers
- C. We learn after verbal communication
- D. That has to be taught
- E. None of the above

3. Which 1 of the following examples is a roadblock to therapeutic communication?

- A. Asking closed-ended questions
- B. Giving advice
- C. Taking notes
- D. Paraphrasing
- E. Gesturing

See the Appendix for the answers.

Remember to use Edge after you finish this chapter to test your knowledge. Directions for how to access Edge, as well as your access code, are located on the inside front cover of this text.

YOUR NOTES

_____

_____

_____

_____

_____

_____

_____

Part 2
Administrative

Chapter 5
Medical Office Administration

This chapter helps you review the general front office duties of a medical practice. The expectation is that you will be familiar with daily office operations, the mail, medical record management, scheduling, bookkeeping, accounting, and banking. The advanced medical assisting knowledge areas also include financial management (payroll, employment forms, and financial summaries), as well as office management (manuals, meetings, equipment, and supplies).

Information regarding medical office administration content within the various national certifying exams may be found in Chapter 1.

 Remember to use Edge after you finish this chapter to test your knowledge. Directions for how to access Edge, as well as your access code, are located on the inside front cover of this text.

Common Abbreviations in Charting and Scheduling

Abbreviation	Meaning
BP	Blood pressure
c/o	Complains of
EHR	Electronic health record

Continued

Abbreviation	Meaning
EMR	Electronic medical record
ESL	English as secondary language
FU or f/u	Follow up
I & D	Incision and drainage
inj	Injection
lab	Laboratory studies
NP	New patient
NS	No show
NSF	Nonsufficient funds
PCP	Primary care provider
pt	Patient
re	Recheck
ref	Referral
Rx	Prescription
S/R	Suture removal
TC	Telephone call
US	Ultrasound
w/o	Without

Preparation for the Day

General Preparation

- **Safety hazard prevention:** Floors should be free of any area rugs and electrical cords, and there should be wide enough areas to have good office traffic flow.
- **Patient records:** Print out the list of patients to be seen the next appointment day. Review the content of

the charts, organize the charts by needs for that day's office visit (OV), and arrange the charts in the order in which the patients are to be seen. One copy of the list of patients is for the physician.

- **Supplies:** Front office area and examination rooms should be checked and replenished with all regular supplies for a given morning or afternoon/evening. Order additional supplies if the medical office supply is low.
- **Community resources:** The office should have an up-to-date listing of local organizations that support patients' health needs, with addresses, telephone numbers, and other contact information. Examples of these resources include legal aid, adult day care, and cardiopulmonary resuscitation (CPR) training.

Clinical Preparation

- **Laboratory equipment:** Perform-quality control tests and log results for certain laboratory machines. This procedure ensures that the equipment is ready for use.
- **Examination rooms:** Prepare these areas for cleanliness and neatness.

Administrative Preparation

- **Answering service/voice mail:** Retrieve, document, and respond to messages left after office hours from the previous day.
- **Office equipment:** Some equipment should be turned on for the day (e.g., copy machines, printers).
- **Reception and front office:** These areas need to be prepared for cleanliness and neatness.

Office Equipment

Space, furnishings, and equipment should incorporate good **ergonomics** (i.e., designed for effectiveness, safety, and comfort).

Facsimile (Fax)

A fax is an electronically scanned copy of a document that is quickly transmitted from 1 location to another over telephone lines. The sender places the document into the fax machine and keys in a destination telephone number to transmit the document. Fax machines also receive documents.

Fax machines need to be located in an area inaccessible to the public to maintain confidentiality of the transmitted information.

- Use only when necessary because violating patient confidentiality is a higher risk.
- Confirmation is received when the transmission is complete.
- Fax machines use designated telephone numbers.
- Use of a cover sheet is required and must state the following:
  - The confidential content, briefly
  - The name of the person to whom it is directed
  - The number of pages being transmitted, including the cover sheet
  - The name and fax number of the sender
- Proper grammar and punctuation must be used.

Photocopier

Creates hard copies of documents (patient insurance cards, patient driver licenses, etc.), which may electronically be added to a patient's electronic medical record (EMR).

Scanner

This electronic equipment converts hard copy documents into a format that a computer can read. It is commonly used in a paperless EMR system medical practice. It may also transmit to an email address.

Computers

Computers are electronic devices for storing and processing data. They can be laptops, desktops, or tablets, or they can be built into medical equipment.

Minicomputer: This functions as a server that stores shared information from other personal computers in a network setting; it is larger than a PC.

Personal computer (PC)/microcomputer: There are 3 types of personal computers commonly used in offices:

- **Desktop:** Most common computer in medical offices. It sits on a desktop at workstations and uses a separate keyboard and mouse or touch pad as the input devices.
- **Laptop (notebook):** A small, portable computer that includes the screen, keyboard, and track pad or track ball to replace the mouse. Laptops weigh just a few pounds. They can operate on battery power or with an AC adapter. Laptops are commonly used in examination rooms to input data on patients into the EMR system.
- **Tablet:** A tablet is a small, flat computer with a touchscreen interface instead of a keyboard and mouse. Tablets are smaller and more portable than laptop computers.

    Computers consist of the following components:

- **Hardware:** This comprises the physical parts of the computer, including the internal pieces.
- **Software:** The installed programs and applications that enable the computer to perform specific tasks and functions. The computer's operating system is the software that starts and controls the computer.

Computer Peripherals

Peripherals, also known as external hardware, include the monitor, keyboard, mouse, printer, and other external devices connected to the computer.

- **Input devices**
    - **Mouse:** Common pointing and scrolling device. It is used for moving the cursor on the computer screen and for moving screen windows. Laptop computers and tablets use trackballs, touch pads, and touch screens as input devices.

- **Keyboard:** Most common input device. It resembles a typewriter, but with the addition of function keys, arrow keys, and a numerical keypad.
- **Output devices**
  - **Monitor:** The television-like screen that shows the computer's open programs. These programs include image software, word processing, information management programs, e-mail, and Internet browsing programs.
  - **Printer:** An output device that produces hard copies, usually on paper, of documents and images from a computer. Laser printers produce the highest quality (resolution), but they are more expensive than ink jet printers.
- **Flash drive**
  - A portable device for temporary storage of files, featuring a built-in Universal Serial Bus (USB) connection that plugs into the computer with a USB port. It is also known as a jump drive, thumb drive, or keychain drive.
- **Health card scanner**
  - This device automates the archiving process and transfers images of medical and insurance cards into a patient's electronic forms.

Network

Two or more computers can be connected to each other in a network. The network allows the sharing of files and information. There are two types of networks in an office setting:

- **Virtual private network (VPN)**
  - This encrypted network uses the Internet to connect two or more computer systems.
  - The security methods used on a VPN ensure data protection.
  - It allows a physician to view confidential patient records from a variety of locations.
- **Local area network (LAN)**
  - A group of computers is linked together either directly with wires or through wireless connections.

- LANs are typically limited to computers within an office or building.
- A LAN is less secure than a VPN.

Computer Terms

Antivirus software: This software is designed to protect a computer from malicious files known as viruses, malware, and spyware. It scans the computer's files and software to destroy and remove the threats to the system. The process is both automatic and manual.

Backup: Action that prevents the loss of files when a hard disk fails. Backup is performed at the end of each business day to store the day's entries.

Bit: This is the smallest unit of data a computer uses to operate or display information. It is either 0 or 1.

Byte: Describes a unit of data having 8 bits. Each byte represents a character such as a letter, number, or symbol.

CD-R: A compact disk used for 1-time data recording and storage.

CD-RW: This compact disk for recording and storage of data can be erased and reused.

CPU (central processing unit): Known as the computer's "brain." This microprocessor interprets and executes program data. It is the most important part of the computer hardware.

Cursor: This is either the arrow seen on the computer screen indicating the position of the mouse or a blinking line indicating the position where the next character keyed will appear in a line of text.

Database: A collection of related information used as a foundation from which information may be retrieved.

Disk drive: This device reads the data or software from a CD or DVD.

DVD: An optical storage disk similar to a CD but capable of holding more data (4.7 to 17 GB, depending on the disk's format).

Firewall: A security system that protects a network or computer from damage by unauthorized users. Such users include hackers attempting to install malicious software or steal information through the Internet.

Gigabyte (GB): A unit of storage representing 1 billion bytes (1,000 megabytes [MB]).

Hard copy: The printout of a document seen on the computer monitor.

HTML (Hypertext Markup Language): This code determines the structure and layout of a Web document.

HTTP (Hypertext Transfer Protocol): The protocol that defines how messages are formatted and transmitted across the Internet. HTTP determines what Web servers and browsers do in response to commands such as entering a search term.

Icons: Small graphic symbols used as visual representations of files, menu functions, or application software.

Menu: Displays the choices of available functions.

Modem: A communication device that allows 1 computer to connect to another or to the Internet through telephone or cable lines.

OCR (optical character recognition): Optical scanning software that converts text on a printed page into text that can be used in word processing software. Without OCR, a scanner scans the printed page as a picture.

Operating system: This software provides the needed instructions (read-only memory [ROM]) to the computer to function. The system starts working when the computer is turned on.

Password: A combination of characters used to verify that you have permission to access a computer or computer system. Passwords are assigned to each employee typically. Management may use the password to track employee computer activity.

Purging: The act of removing unnecessary old data from a hard drive or disk drive.

RAM (random access memory): Temporary memory a program uses to speed up its retrieval of operating data. Computers with more RAM can run more complicated software programs more quickly.

ROM (read-only memory): Permanent, unchangeable basic operating instructions. The computer needs these instructions to function.

Terabyte (TB): The term used to represent 1,000 gigabytes (GB).

USB (Universal Serial Bus): The standardized cable and plug used to connect computer peripherals to computers.

WAN (wide area network): A network of computers spread across a larger geographical area than a LAN. WANs are usually connected by telephone lines.

YOUR NOTES

_____

_____

_____

_____

_____

_____

_____

Sending and Receiving Mail

Annotate: To underline or highlight significant words and key points. Annotations can identify anything in the mail that needs a response, or they can be reminders, comments, and suggestions for action.

Postage meter: A machine that prints postage, cancellation marks, and dates directly onto envelopes or onto package labels. Most postage meters are connected to scales to weigh the piece. Offices must purchase the amount of postage each machine can print, which is programmed into the machine by the U.S. Postal Service.

Physician's personal mail: If mail has been marked "personal," it should be placed unopened on the physician's desk in an easily visible area (e.g., on top of the day's charts).

Types of Mail

First-Class Mail:
- Weighs 13 oz or less
- Maximum size for a large envelope: 15 inches long by 12 inches high by ¾-inch thick.
- Maximum size for package (box): 108 inches in combined length and distance around the thickest part
- Number 10 envelopes, postcards, green diamond bordered envelopes
- Must be rectangular
- 2- to 3-day delivery

Priority Mail: Same as first class; maximum weight is 70 lb. The package can be tracked.

Parcel Post (standard post): Maximum weight is 70 lb, with 130 inches in combined length and distance around the thickest part; 2- to 8-day delivery. This is used for books, catalogues, and general merchandise.

Certified Mail: Guarantees the delivery of an item. On delivery, the postal carrier obtains the signature of the receiver. The words printed on paper (e.g., contracts, birth certificates) have more value than the paper they are printed on.

Registered Mail: In addition to delivery confirmation, registered mail includes insurance and additional security services for high-dollar-value or irreplaceable items (e.g., jewels, medications). The item is placed in a lockbox that is signed by each postal worker as it changes hands on the way to its destination.

Express Mail: Next day delivery if sent by 5 p.m. Mail can weigh up to 70 lb; there is proof of delivery, and the item may be insured for up to $100.

Special Delivery: Delivery is as soon as possible once the mail reaches the local post office for final delivery.

Private delivery services: Companies such as Federal Express, United Parcel Service (UPS), DHL, and smaller courier services offer faster and more secure delivery than the U.S. Postal Service.

Medical Records

Record Ownership

The treating physician owns the record material, whereas the patient owns the information in the record.

- Records are used to provide:
  - Best medical care
  - Statistics
  - Liability case defense (good documentation is part of risk management)
  - Quality of treatment assessment

Record Retention

Records are kept for 7 to 10 years for adults and for 7 to 10 years from reaching the age of majority for minors.

Active files: Most often, the patient has been treated within the last 6 months to 3 years (depending on the practice specialty).

Inactive files: The patient has not been treated within the last 6 months to 3 years (depending on the practice specialty).

Closed files: The patient is not expected to return (moving, age limit in pediatrics, death).

Release of records with authorization: This allows the sending of record copies to the designated physician.

Release of records without authorization: These records may be released because of a life-threatening circumstance (e.g., unconscious patient).

Medical or Accounting Records Error Correction

* Draw a line through the error.
* Write the correct data above or below the error; add the date and time, and initial it.
* Do not attempt to erase or use correction fluid or tape; all medical records are legal documents.

Record Organization

Problem-Oriented Medical Record (POMR)

* Problems are numbered.
* Includes database
  * **Demographics** (name, address, date of birth [DOB], health insurance, contact information)
  * Profile history, chief complaint (cc), case conceptualization
  * Past assessments and test results; treatment plan: procedures, medications
  * Instructions; progress notes; continuous care notes

Source-Oriented Medical Record (SOMR)

* The record is divided into sections (e.g., laboratory, progress notes, physical examinations [PEs], consultation reports).
* Each section is arranged in chronological order; the most recent document is on top in each section.

Subjective Objective Assessment Plan (SOAP)

SOAP is a common method used to document information about a patient during the OV:

- **Subjective:** Symptoms not seen, heard, or measured. This information is given by the patient. If it is not volunteered by the patient, then it is not known.
- **Objective:** Signs read in test results that are heard, measured, or observed.
- **Assessment:** Findings that combine subjective and objective information into a probable diagnosis.
- **Plan:** Treatment based on the diagnosis (e.g., medication, further tests, education, therapy).

Electronic Records

Electronic Medical Record (EMR)

- Software is used to create and use records. The goal is a paperless office.
- EMR usually works with the practice management (financial) functions of the office.
- It includes the patient's demographics: insurance and billing information; previous medical history; current condition, treatment, and progress.
- Advantages
  - Efficiency: It can reduce medical errors.
  - Accessibility: Security is ensured through the use of a user password.
  - Speed: Patient information is available quickly.
  - Productivity: Providers may access patient information.
  - Legible: Information is typed into a medical record.
- Disadvantages
  - Initial cost
  - Time investment (training)
  - Operational tasks

Electronic Health Record (EHR)

- EMR information about a patient is created and managed in a format that allows the information to be shared nationally with other authorized health-care provider computer systems because of its interoperability.
- This is a fully integrated system: patient demographics, lab results, scheduling, health-care and history records, all forms of communication, medication(s), etc.
- **Point-of-Care:** All clinical staff may enter patient information into the record.

Filing Systems

- **Direct filing:** Alphabetical
  - First indexing unit: Last name (surname)
  - Second indexing unit: First name
  - Third indexing unit: Middle initial or name
  - Fourth indexing unit: Titles, suffixes (e.g., Jr., Dr., Atty.)
- **Indirect filing:** Numerical
  - It uses a terminal digit. The filing order is read from right to left.
  - It provides the highest confidentiality.
  - It is used in large clinics and hospitals.
- **Color coding:** Easy retrieval. This lessens the number of misfiles.
- **Subjective:** Topics are arranged alphabetically.
- **Tickler:** This chronological file is arranged by date and time set as a reminder to perform tasks.

Paper Chart Filing Procedures

Inspecting: Making sure the physician has indicated that the chart was reviewed and the required actions were done

Indexing: Determining where each document needs to be filed within a chart

Coding: Highlighting the name/subject of a document

Sorting: Using the alphabetical method to subdivide the documents to be filed in charts

Storing: Placing the document in the proper chart, within the proper section of that chart, and in the proper chronological order

---

YOUR NOTES

_____

_____

_____

_____

_____

_____

_____

Scheduling

Physician preference: The first consideration in creating the practice's scheduling system is the physician's preference.

Matrix: The blocked-off time slots during which no appointments (OVs) are scheduled.

• It is completed before scheduling any appointments.

Buffer times: Certain time slots are left unfilled until that day in the office.

• More are needed on Mondays and Fridays.

Missed OVs: Document in the medical record and make a notation in the day's schedule planner.

Cancellations: Document in the medical record and make a notation in the day's schedule planner.

Confirmation: Office personnel call or text scheduled patients to confirm their upcoming appointments. Performing this task helps to ensure the office that the patient will not miss an OV and serves as a patient reminder.

Types of Scheduling Systems

Open hours (tidal)	• 1st come, 1st served • Common scheduling format in urgent care centers
Wave	• Usually 4 patients seen per hour • All scheduled for top of hour, seen in order of arrival
Modified wave	• In 1-hour frame; 2 patients given own specific time, 2 told to arrive at same time (e.g., 10:30)
Clustering (grouping)	• Same type of office visits all scheduled in same block (certain day, a.m. or p.m.) • Higher efficiency and speed
Double booking	• 2 or more patients scheduled with same physician at same time, overbooking • Not good schedule planning; causes many delays
Stream (time specified)	• Each patient given own specific time • Most common method of scheduling
Advanced booking	• Commonly done with established patients • Involves scheduling weeks or months in advance

Bookkeeping and Accounting

Bookkeeping

Bookkeeping is the day-by-day detailed recording of business transactions (debits, credits, disbursements). It is a part of the accounting process.

Balance: The difference between the fee charged and the payment made toward that fee

Charge: Fee incurred for a provided service

Credit: Payment made toward a debt (debit) owed

Credit adjustment: The dollar amount written off (the office will not collect it)

- It is the difference between the amount charged and the amount allowed by the insurance carrier.
- It may be the result of provider participation with the patient's insurance plan.
- It may be the result of discounts given because of special circumstances.

Credit balance: An overpayment, often when payments are made from different sources

Debit: Debt, money owed for services charged

Disbursement: Money that is sent from a business as payment for what is owed to others (e.g., rent, leased equipment, medical supplies)

General journal (day sheet): Detailed chronological record of services given, charges, and receipts

Liabilities: Monies (debts) owed to others (e.g., rent, phone, equipment leases)

Posting: The act of recording information (noting payment in day sheet, account ledger, etc.)

Superbill, Encounter form, Charge slip, Statement:
- This contains diagnoses, procedures, and services performed, patient insurance information, provider information, and signature.
- It may be used to bill insurance.

Transaction: Any financial exchange, such as services provided for a fee

Accounting

Accounting is the process of keeping summaries made from the daily bookkeeping entries (credits, debits, disbursements) to provide the office with financial information about the business.

Accounts payable: Monies owed by the business (e.g., rent and supplies).

Accounts receivable: Monies owed to the business from patients.

Accounts receivable control: The total money owed to the practice at close of each business day.

Accrual basis: Sold items are considered income, even if they have not been paid for at the time.

Cash basis: Charges are entered as income once payment is received for services; medical offices use this system.

Double entry: A method of accounting based on the following equation: **Assets = Liabilities + Capital (owner equity).** Entries are listed twice, based on each transaction. Certified Public Accountants (CPAs) and specially trained bookkeepers use this form of accounting. It detects errors easily.

* *Assets* are possessions of value (office equipment, inventory, account receivables, bank accounts, etc.).
* *Liabilities* are debts owed by the office (e.g., lease payments, loan payments, various insurance premium payments, payroll, medical and office supply bills).
* *Equities* are the rights to the assets, the portion of the assets that is paid for.

Patient account ledger: Used to record and maintain an account of each patient's financial transactions (charges and payments). The ledger can either be a paper or computer accounting system.

Single-entry system: Method of accounting in its simplest form. It is not self-balancing because simple summaries are listed once only for the patient ledgers, general ledger, and checkbook. Finding entry errors is most difficult with this system.

Banking

ABA number: Identifies the exact bank location of a check's origin; it is located on the upper right side of a check.

Bank draft: A check written by a bank against its funds in another bank.

Cashier's check (treasurer's check): This is the bank's own check and is signed by a bank representative.

Certified check: The payer's own check, officially stamped by the bank. This guarantees the availability of funds by setting the check amount in the account aside; the payee is assured of payment.

Limited check: This has a time limit (90 days) or is pre-printed for maximum amount limit.

Magnetic ink character recognition (MICR) code: A magnetic ink code is printed across the bottom of a check; it is used by the bank for sorting checks. A part of the code is the ABA routing number.

Money order: A type of guaranteed payment is purchased in cash for a small fee. Money orders are a safe way to send money, especially if an individual does not have a checking account. They may be purchased for a small fee through the U.S. Postal Service, banks, and some stores.

Online payment: A form of banking available through the Internet. An online bill paying account is established with a bank or other business. Payment for a single bill is accepted directly. Payment for a monthly bill is made automatically when the bill is due.

* Banking is available 24 hours a day.
* Transactions are accomplished in seconds.

Overdraft, nonsufficient funds (NSF): Money in the checking account is too low to cover the check amount. This is also referred to as a bounced check.

Payee: The person, practice, or company to whom the check is written (payable).

Payer: The person who signs the check to release the money to the payee.

Power of attorney: In terms of banking, this written authorization grants a person the legal right to handle the financial matters of another person.

Third-party check: A check not originally written to the party receiving it. The check is written by an unknown party to the payee; therefore, if it were to become an overdraft (bounce) on cashing or deposit, it would become very difficult to track the originator of the check for payment.

• Only accept insurance checks written to the patient as payment.

Traveler's check: Checks purchased at face value from an issuing bank for a small fee. The checks are protected against theft or loss, and they are commonly used when traveling to where personal checks may not be accepted.

• Available in small or large denominations: $10, $20, $50, $100

Endorsement: An endorsement is a signature on the back of a check that may or may not have more information noted below the signature. The name of the last endorser of the check shows who last received the money. The common types of endorsement are

• **Blank:** Most common, signature only
• **Restrictive:** "For deposit only" stamped on check back (immediately on receipt)
• **Limited (special):** "Pay to the order of" followed by signature of patient paying
• **Qualified:** "Without recourse," used by lawyers accepting checks by clients
• **Voucher check:** With detachable part giving payee additional information (i.e., payroll checks)

Financial Management

Accounts payable: Money owed by the medical practice. These are operating expenses.

Accounts receivable: Money owed to the medical practice or the medical practice's income.

Age analysis (age of accounts receivable): Age analysis tracks the age of debts by assigning accounts receivables into categories, such as the length of time from the date of service.

Total Accounts Receivable	Amount That Is 1–3 Months Old	Amount That Is 4–6 Months Old	Amount That Is 7–9 Months Old	Amount That Is 10–12 Months Old
$425.00	$75.00	$280.00	$70.00	$0.00

Balance sheet: A record of the total assets, liabilities, and capital of a business for a specific date.

Bank statement: The record of all checking account (checkbook) financial transactions.

* It displays processed deposits and checks, interest earned, and service charges over a specific time frame: first of month to last day of given month.

Checkbook: A book of blank checks with a log (register) for recording written checks and deposits.

* Summaries of receipts called deposits are recorded in the checkbook's log.
* Bills (accounts payable) are paid from this checking account.

Disbursement record (journal): A summary of monies paid over a specific time period (a part of accounts payable management).

* It shows each amount paid out, date and check number, and category of payment (e.g., office supplies, medical supplies).

Payroll record: Part of accounts payable management. It is kept separate from other payables because of necessary tracking of each employee's gross income and withholdings.

Petty cash: Part of accounts payable management. These monies are used to pay for small, unexpected office expenses and are kept separate from the business office accounting. The petty cash account usually has no more than $200 in it at any time. It is funded by the office's own checking account.

Reconciliation: Balancing a checkbook with the bank statement:

1. Start with the bank statement balance.
2. Add deposits not seen on the bank statement.
3. Subtract outstanding checks not seen on the statement.
4. Add the remaining dollar amount; this should be the checkbook balance.

Financial Summaries

Accounts receivable ratio: This ratio measures the speed at which outstanding balances are paid; it begins from the day billing is sent to when payment is received.

Cash flow statement: Displays all expenses and income activity within time frame, plus depreciation and liabilities. It shows the account balance and cash on hand from start to end date. It reflects amount of money available to cover expenses, to invest, or to take profits.

Collection ratio: This calculation measures the effectiveness of the office billing system (e.g., 97% of billed amount is paid).

Statement of income and expenses: Profit and loss. This is a summary of all income and expenses for a time period.

Trial balance: This checks the accuracy of accounts to ensure the books are in balance.

- Accounts receivable control should match total of all patients' accounts receivable ledgers.
- The total amount of the checks written should equal the total of disbursements (the expense columns in the general ledger).

Office Management

Manuals

Office policy manual: Information for employees regarding office operations, policies, and regulations, as well as workplace laws. The manual should always be read and periodically reviewed as necessary by employees and agencies.

- The manual can include sections on
  - Mission statement (usually stated at the beginning of the manual)
  - Sexual harassment
  - Confidentiality
  - Patients' rights
  - Office's organizational chart
  - Position interviewing, hiring, and firing
  - Sick leave and vacation
  - Personnel evaluations
  - Dress code
  - Staff meetings
  - Workflow
  - Office maintenance

Procedure ("how to") manual: This manual contains descriptions of situations and tasks.

- The manual can include sections on
  - Job descriptions (e.g., clinical medical assistant, licensed practical nurse, receptionist)
  - Step-by-step guide for each procedure in a given position
  - Situation handling

Office Meetings

Staff meetings are held weekly or monthly as needed or preferred to correct situations and to share information affecting office practice, performance, and procedures.

Meeting agenda: Focuses meeting by using an orderly list of items to be discussed

Meeting minutes: Official record of meeting proceedings

- Assist attendees with decisions or suggestions for next meeting
- Must be approved by motion
- Contents: name of committee; date, time, and type of meeting; members present; items of business discussed

(no summaries); motions made, approved, and rejected; adjournment time; next meeting date if any

Office Equipment

Inventory

The inventory is a list of in-stock supply items and pieces of equipment. Ordering, storage, and usage of equipment and supplies are tracked using an inventory system.

- Office equipment is listed by date of purchase, serial number, service dates, and warranties.
- Reasons for listing:
  - Stocking: To avoid running too low on important supplies
  - Depreciation: A 5-year period for large, durable equipment pieces (for tax purposes)
  - Damage or theft: Reporting to manufacturers or police
- Inventory of equipment and supplies include the following:
  - General supplies (e.g., toilet tissue and paper towels)
  - Administrative supplies (e.g., stationery, copier/fax toner, pens, and highlighters)
  - Clinical supplies (e.g., table paper, instruments, and tongue depressors)
  - Capital equipment (e.g., computers, copier, examination tables, and an electrocardiogram machine)

Equipment Maintenance

Maintenance agreements: These are made for periodic upkeep (cleaning) of computers, copiers, fax machines, autoclaves, microscopes, and other equipment.

Replacement: This usually occurs as part of a maintenance agreement. The office pays for the replaced part, not the labor.

Warranty: This document is sent to the manufacturer on receipt of the equipment.

- It ensures replacement of defective parts and equipment.
- It usually has a replacement period up to 1 year from purchase.

Service contracts: These agreements provide repairs when called on for a contracted time period after the warranty has expired.

Receiving of Supplies Ordered

Invoice: May be included with the delivered items. It displays the amount due for each item.

Packing slip: Included with the product delivery. It describes the enclosed items.

Statement: A bill for all invoices delivered in 1 month.

Payroll and Forms

Employee payroll detail must be kept for at least 4 years for Internal Revenue Service (IRS) purposes.

Gross: The total amount earned in a pay period before deductions are made.

Net: The earned income after deductions are made: "take home pay."

Salary: Fixed amount paid to an employee regardless of hours worked in pay period.

Wages: Earnings paid based on an hourly rate.

• If working more than 40 hours per week, 1.5 times the hourly wage is paid for each overtime hour.

Deductions: Employers are required to withhold the following from employee earnings:

• Federal income tax
• Social security tax; referred to as FICA (Federal Insurance Contributions Act)
• Medicare tax
• State tax (depending on location)

EIN (Employer tax ID number): Each employer must have this number for reporting federal taxes.

Federal withholding tax: Money withheld from an employee's gross earnings to pay federal income tax. The employer deposits this money into a tax liability account.

Employee Forms

W2: Federal tax form given to employees by January 31. It details the previous year's wage detail (gross income total, various withheld taxes).

W4: Employees withholding allowance certificate. It is completed by a new employee before the first pay period; the number of tax exemptions (individuals who depend on the employee's financial support) is noted here. This document is kept in the employer's personnel file and is updated annually or any time changes occur.

Employer Forms and Payments

W3: A transmittal of Wage and Tax Statements that lists the employer's name, address, and EIN. In addition, it documents a summary of employee earnings, FICA, and federal taxes withheld. The employer sends it to the Social Security Administration with government copies of employee W2 forms.

FICA (Federal Insurance and Contributions Act): This is the Social Security and Medicare percentage of income withheld from employee paychecks.

- **Deposit requirements:** The employer is required to deposit the FICA percentage to a federal deposit account in a Federal Reserve or authorized bank each month.
- **Dollar amount due:** The employer pays the federal tax withheld plus double the FICA tax withheld.

Form 940 FUTA (Federal Unemployment Tax Act): Percentage of an employee's paycheck paid by the employer toward the unemployment fund. This is not deducted from the employee's gross income. It is paid annually to the IRS.

Form 941: Employer's quarterly federal tax return to report federal income tax and FICA taxes withheld from employee paychecks. It is due within 1 month after each quarter: April 30, July 31, October 31, and January 31.

Sample Certification Test Questions

Now that you have studied this chapter, here are some sample certification test questions for you.

1. An example of the demographic information in a medical record is
   A. School sports physical examination outcomes
   B. Date of birth (DOB)
   C. Chief complaint
   D. Chest x-ray result
   E. Laboratory reports

2. When a medical facility uses the numerical filing system, which of the following is needed?
   A. An alpha cross reference
   B. A chronological reference
   C. A tickler file reference
   D. Color code reference
   E. None of the above

3. Which of the following office equipment is inventoried for depreciation?
   A. Examination table paper
   B. Syringes
   C. Letterhead paper
   D. Autoclave
   E. Stethoscope

See the Appendix for the answers.

Remember to use Edge after you finish this chapter to test your knowledge. Directions for how to access Edge, as well as your access code, are located on the inside front cover of this text.

Chapter 6

Medical Insurance, Billing, and Coding

Put simply, a medical practice is a business and therefore must charge for services provided to its patients and collect payment. Health insurance is meant to offset the rising costs of health care through monetary benefits that cover the expenses of preemptive care, illness, or injury. Correct documentation of the provided services and claim submission to the insurance carriers ensure that the medical practice receives prompt processing and payment. To document the services correctly, all medical providers use a common coding language to describe necessary care of a patient resulting from illness, a condition, family history, injury, health maintenance, or preventive treatment.

Consequently, this chapter begins by examining the language of insurance. Detail is provided on the types of insurance, managed care, and government plans. This explanation is followed by an introduction to both Current Procedural Terminology (CPT) and International Classification of Diseases (ICD) coding. Finally, billing and fee collection are covered.

Information regarding insurance, billing, and coding content within the various national certifying exams may be found in Chapter 1.

Remember to use Edge after you finish this chapter to test your knowledge. Directions for how to access Edge, as well as your access code, are located on the inside front cover of this text.

Common Insurance and Billing Abbreviations

Abbreviation	Meaning
CMS	Centers for Medicare & Medicaid Services (administers funding)
E&M	Evaluation and management (CPT office visit procedure codes)
EIN	Employer identification number
EOB	Explanation of benefits (sent by insurance carrier to provider; gives breakdown of reimbursement for services billed)
EOMB	Explanation of Medicare benefits (sent to provider; gives breakdown of reimbursement for services billed
EPSDT	Early and periodic screening, diagnosis, and treatment
IRS	Internal Revenue Service
LOS	Length of stay
MEDI/MEDI	Term used for Medicare and Medicaid coverage
NSF	Nonsufficient funds
PF	Problem focused
PIN	Provider identification number
RA	Remittance advice (sent by Medicaid to provider; gives breakdown of reimbursement for services billed)
SOF	Signature on file; signed copy authorizing claim submission and direct payment to provider
UR	Utilization review; examination of services provided; performed by unaffiliated group to determine medical necessity

CPT, Current Procedural Terminology.

Health-Care Coverage Terminology

Allowed charge: The maximum dollar amount an insurance carrier will cover for a provided service.

Assignment of benefits: The patient authorizes the insurance carrier to pay the physician directly. The patient's signature is required. Assignment is automatically in place if the provider is a participating (PAR) provider with the insurance carrier.

Beneficiary: The beneficiaries are the subscriber and eligible person(s) named by the subscriber (policyholder) to receive insurance benefits.

Birthday rule: Determines which insurance company is billed 1st (primary). The rule is enforced if the covered individual is the beneficiary of more than 1 health insurance policy.

Capitation: Fixed dollar amount paid by the insurance company to the PAR provider, usually 1 to 2 times per month, for each enrolled patient. The number and types of services provided to a patient do not influence the dollar amount paid.

Clearinghouse: Used to scrutinize claims for correctness after they have been electronically transmitted from the health-care provider but before the insurance carrier receives them. A clearinghouse may be part of the software package used by the provider.

Coordination of benefits: Limits benefits to 100% of the cost of service when there is more than 1 insurance carrier used for coverage. The primary insurance pays the required contractual amount; the secondary insurance pays the remainder of the allowable amount.

Diagnosis-related group (DRG): Determines payment for a hospital claim under Medicare Part A. This is arrived at by using a system based on a patient's primary diagnosis, the course of treatment, and length of stay in a hospital. A finalized DRG claim is then submitted to Medicare.

Direct billing: Term used to describe the electronic claim submission transmitted from the provider to the insurance carrier for processing. No vendor is used to examine claims for correctness.

Electronic claims: Preferred method of claim submission; reduces time in mailing and claim processing. Transmission is from computer to computer.

Fee profile: The given physician's usual charges for various procedures compiled over time.

Fee schedule: The preset dollar amount an insurance company allows for each service or procedure (e.g., physician charges $75 for 99213; insurance fee schedule allows $68 for 99213).

Fiscal agent (fiscal intermediary): A company that processes insurance claims on behalf of a health insurance plan. It is used by Medicare and Medicaid in each state.

Formulary: Listing of insurance-covered prescription medications. The purpose is to lower costs through use of generic drugs.

Guarantor (sometimes referred to as the insured or subscriber): This individual is financially responsible for payment for himself or herself or for a family member.

Nonparticipating (NON-PAR) provider: A provider of services who does not have an agreement with an insurance carrier. The provider expects full payment from the patient for billed services.

Participating or member (PAR) provider: A physician who has an agreement or is contracted with an insurance carrier to accept the company's allowed charge as 100% payment. The physician writes off the difference between the physician's usual fee and the allowed charge.

Preauthorization: The approval given from an insurance company for service (e.g., procedure, therapy, surgery, hospitalization) resulting from medical necessity.

Precertification: The process used by an insurance company to determine coverage for a specific service.

Premium: The dollar amount paid (by patient and/or employer) for insurance coverage.

- Factors that lower the cost of the premium:
  1. Deductible: Out-of-pocket money before insurance makes payment
  2. Copayment: Set amount patient pays for each office visit (e.g., $10, $15)
  3. Co-insurance: Percentage that patient pays for each office visit (usually 20%)

Professional courtesy: This represents a reduced charge or free service to a professional associate.

Referral: A directive, executed by the primary care physician (PCP), for the patient to seek specialized care from a preferred provider. This is commonly used for managed care plans.

Resource-Based Relative Value Scale (RBRVS): Used by Medicare to determine the fee schedule for Medicare Part B. The dollar amounts are based on factors involving the procedure performed and the provider's geographic location.

Rider: An addition made to an insurance policy. It usually stipulates exclusions for preexisting chronic conditions and/or procedures for a specific time (e.g., 1st 6 months).

Risk withhold: A portion of the capitation payment to a provider that is withheld until the end of the year or defined fiscal year. This is done to create incentive for efficient care.

Subscriber or policyholder: This is the primary person covered by insurance.

Third-party payer (administrator): This is usually the paying insurance carrier.

UCR: Used to determine payable insurance benefits for performed procedures:

U: Usual fees a physician charges for most frequently used procedures

C: Customary fees charged by physicians in the same geographic area and specialty

R: Reasonable fees that are justifiable when the usual procedure is more complicated

YOUR NOTES

_____

_____

_____

_____

_____

_____

_____

Types of Health Insurance

Type	Description
Major medical (catastrophic insurance)	• Assists in paying for unexpected medical expenses (hospitalizations) • High deductible helps keep premium cost low
Workers' Compensation	• Employer medical and disability insurance for employee death, injury, illness on the job or related to the job • Physician sends "First Report of Occupational Injury" within 72 hours of patient's 1st visit • Patient not billed
Self-insured plan	• Employer-provided staffed health facility on site to cover employee needs • Drug testing, physical examinations, special job-related testing

Type	Description
Group	• Offered by employers to employee groups • Low premiums • All employees may join in lieu of physical examination • Typically uses managed care plans such as HMOs • Usually no physical examination required to join
Consolidated Omnibus Budget Reconciliation Act (COBRA)	• Up to 18 months health plan coverage offered by employers of 20 or more qualified employees and their dependents • Qualification(s) is/are: • Divorce from spouse • Employee death • Employee termination • End of dependent benefits related to age maturity
Health savings account (HSA)	• Uses a savings account from which deductible is paid • Preventive care at no cost; no deductible applied • High-deductible health insurance plan • Monthly premiums based on age, geographic area, and deductible • No taxes on withdrawals if used for medical expenses
Individual	• Coverage purchased by individual • Usually requires physical examination to qualify • High premium cost • Medigap, crossover: A supplemental policy purchased by an individual more than 65 years old to pay Medicare deductibles and 20% co-insurance
Indemnity	• Specific dollar amount paid for each service • Patient pays any remaining amount due • Works on a fee-for-service basis

HMO, health maintenance organization.

Managed Care

- The patient's choice of physician is limited to PAR providers.
- The patient's access is limited to PAR facilities.
- The patient selects a PCP.
- Utilization review (UR) by the plan evaluates the proposed or current patient treatment.
- It may require the use of referrals from the PCP to specialists.
- It includes preventive health-care medicine.

Managed Care Organizations (MCOs)

Plan	Description
Health maintenance organization (HMO)	• Staff model: Salaried MDs work only for plan • Network model: • MD groups are contracted • MD may also contract with other health insurance organizations • MD refers patients to PAR providers only • Patient pays copayments • Patient is restricted to using a PCP belonging to the network
Preferred provider organization (PPO)	• Patient can use services in and out of network • MD rewarded for using in-network services only • Patient pays deductibles and co-insurance
Exclusive provider organization (EPO)	• In-network coverage only • Employer must contract only with EPO • Out-of-network coverage is available for emergencies or travel outside of service area only
Independent practice association (IPA)	• Formally organized groups of MDs working independently • MDs paid by subscriber (policyholder) funds • Partial payment of allowable risk withhold paid at end of fiscal year

Plan	Description
Point of service (POS)	• Combine HMO and PPO plans • Patient must designate a PCP • Out-of-network coverage • Patient has a higher deductible and co-insurance

PAR, participating; PCP, primary care physician.

YOUR NOTES

_____

_____

_____

_____

_____

_____

Government Health Plans

Plan	Description
Medicare	• Federally funded • For individuals in the following categories: more than 65 years old with a minimum of 10 years of Medicare-approved employment; disabled; with end-stage kidney disease; kidney donors; or retired railway employees • **Part A:** Automatic enrollment, inpatient coverage, new deductible to meet for each hospital admission • **Part B:** Voluntary enrollment, adds outpatient coverage, yearly deductible, monthly premium due • **Part C:** Medicare managed care plans; replace Part A and B • **Part D:** Prescription (Rx) plans

Continued

Plan	Description
Medicaid	• Federally and state funded • Title XIX; for medically indigent (low-income individuals and families) • Last health-care coverage to bill if there is other coverage • If patient is treated, assignment is automatic, and allowed payment is considered payment in full • Cannot bill patient for covered services
Children's Health Insurance Program (CHIP)	• Federally and state funded • Managed by individual states
TRICARE	• Federally funded • Covers families of military active personnel and retirees • Dependents and surviving spouses are covered if the veteran was killed in active duty • Costs vary and are based on the plan selected, enrollment date, and if currently active, retired, or medically retired
CHAMPVA	• Federally funded • Covers disabled veterans • Covers families of veterans with total, permanent service-related disabilities and those who died in line of duty

HMO, health maintenance organization.

Related Insurance

Plan	Description
Liability	• If injury occurs on site: covers homeowner and/or business • If injury results from vehicle accident: covers occupants
Life	• Pays beneficiary a set dollar amount in the event of the policyholder's death

YOUR NOTES

_____

_____

_____

_____

_____

_____

Coding

Each reason a patient comes to a medical office results in at least 1 diagnostic code and 1 procedure code. The procedure coding manuals (CPT and Healthcare Common Procedure Coding System [HCPCS]) and the diagnostic coding manual (ICD) are updated annually.

Procedure Coding

The HCPCS is used in the United States. It is based on the American Medical Association's CPT. The procedures and services performed in a medical office are translated into numbers and alphanumeric codes.

HCPCS includes 2 currently used levels:

- Level I codes are known as CPT codes (numeric).
- Level II codes are known as national codes (alphanumeric).

Level I Categories

Level I coding is divided into 3 categories:

- Category I
  - Procedures that are consistent with current medical practice and are widely performed

- In the main body of the CPT manual
- Consisting of 5 digits
- Category II
  - Supplementary tracking codes that are used for performance measures
  - Use optional; not a substitute for category I
  - Consists of 4 digits followed by the letter "F"
- Category III
  - Temporary codes for emerging technology, services, and procedures
  - Retired within 5 years if not adopted as category I
  - Payment for these services based on policies of payers and not on a yearly fee schedule
  - Consists of 5 characters followed by 4 digits followed by the letter "T"

The CPT Manual Organization

- Brief listing of symbols and modifiers
- Place-of-Service codes
- Introduction to the manual
- Illustrated anatomical and procedural review

The following is the tabular (numeric) index: You are led to this section from the alphabetic section to finalize the proper code to use.

- Evaluation and Management (E&M) Services Guidelines and Codes
- Anesthesia Guidelines and Codes
- Surgery Guidelines and Codes
- Radiology Guidelines and Codes
- Pathology and Laboratory Guidelines and Codes
- Medicine Guidelines and Codes
- Category II Codes
- Category III Codes
- Appendices
- Alphabetic index: This is where you begin to search for a procedure code.

There are 6 helpful ways to begin the search for a code within the alphabetical index:

1. Procedure or service performed (e.g., incisions, electro-cardiogram [ECG])
2. Anatomic site or organ (e.g., abdomen, kidney)
3. Condition (e.g., lesions, adhesions, tumors)
4. Synonym (e.g., throat = pharynx; heart = cardiac)
5. Eponym; the proper name of the inventor or discoverer (e.g., Colles fracture)
6. Abbreviation (e.g., EEG, ECG, MRI)

The following table shows the 6 main tabular sections of the CPT manual.

Section	Description
Evaluation and management (E&M)	**99202–99499** 3 main components: • **History:** HPI (history of present illness), PFSH (patient, family, social history) • **Examination:** ROS (review of systems): 1 or more body systems • **Decision making** (straightforward to highly complex) 3 contributing components: • Time, counseling, coordination of care
Anesthesiology	**00100–01999, 99100–99140**
Surgery (the largest section)	**10004–69990**
Radiology	**70010–79999**
Pathology and laboratory	**80047–89398, 0001U–0222U**
Medicine (except anesthesiology)	**90281–99199, 99500–99607**

Examination Hint

The 1st number of a listed procedure code refers to a specific section of the coding manual. On the examination, you can use the section number to determine whether the code correctly matches the definition.

Example: For 30150, a correct match is "rhinectomy, partial." An incorrect match is "office or other outpatient visit."

Unlisted procedure or service: Usually identified by the **"99"** in the last 2 characters. The procedure or service must be performed by physicians or qualified health-care professionals and not listed in the CPT code manual. When reporting this service code, a **special report** must accompany the submission.

Modifier: Made up of 2 characters that provide additional information for the procedure code identified. A modifier does not change the code meaning, but it identifies any special circumstance that should be considered by the claim recipient. It is similar to an adjective used to describe a noun. A complete listing of modifiers is found in Appendix A of the CPT manual. The following are examples of modifiers and their description:

22 Increased procedural services
26 Professional component
52 Reduced services
54 Surgical care only; another physician provided preoperative and postoperative services
56 Preoperative management only

A complete listing of modifiers with definitions is located in Appendix A of the CPT manual.

Place-of-Service Codes

These codes should be used on professional claims to specify where each service/procedure is performed. These codes consist of 2 numbers. The following are examples:

02 Telehealth: Services performed or received through a telecommunication system

03 School: Facility where the primary purpose is education

11 Office: Where the health-care professional routinely provides health examinations, diagnosis, and treatment; not a hospital, skilled nursing facility, military facility, community health-care center, public health clinic, or intermediate-care facility

24 Ambulatory Surgical Center: A free-standing facility where surgical and diagnostic services are provided on an ambulatory basis; not a physician's office

A complete listing of these codes is located at the beginning of the CPT manual.

CPT Terminology

Bundling: One CPT code is used in place of multiple available codes to identify a procedure fully.

Consultation: This consists of the advice and/or opinion of a physician asked for by another physician.

Down code: A less complicated and/or simpler management code is substituted for a more complicated and/or complex code when irregularities are found within a submitted claim. The result is lower financial reimbursement by an insurance carrier to the provider.

Established patient: A patient who has received service within the past 3 years from a particular medical provider or that provider's medical practice.

New patient: A patient who has not received service in the past 3 years from a particular physician or that physician's medical practice.

Referral: A written form, verbal notification by telephone, or other communication that is needed to send a patient from 1 physician (usually a PCP) to another. The form in which the referral is accomplished depends on the insurance carrier.

Up code: An insurance claim purposely coded to the next highest reimbursable code that does not have proper documentation to support its use.

Healthcare Common Procedure Coding System

- Level II codes.
- These codes were developed by the Health Care Financing Administration (HCFA; now Centers for Medicare & Medicaid Services [CMS]).
- Their use is required for Medicare and Medicaid patient care.
- These codes are used by providers to describe specific items and services provided in health care delivery (e.g., laboratory, pathology, pharmaceutical, supplies and durable medical equipment, and ambulance services) that are not covered by CPT level I codes.
- Alphanumeric: Each code begins with a letter.

YOUR NOTES

_____

_____

_____

_____

_____

_____

Diagnostic Coding

International Classification of Disease

- The World Health Organization (WHO) develops and uses the ICD code system to compile data on morbidity and mortality. It is the classification standard for established diseases and other health conditions.
- Codes are made up of characters (numbers and letters). Three characters make up a coding category, which may

be further subdivided or used if it cannot be further sub-divided. Subcategories are made up of 4, 5, 6, or 7 char-acters to provide greater detail. For a code to be valid, it must be coded to the full number of characters required for that code.

The U.S. Federal Government's Adaptions of the ICD

* The *International Classification of Diseases, Tenth Revision, Procedure Coding System (ICD-10-PCS)* is the comprehen-sive manual used for **inpatient procedural codes.** The CMS agency is responsible for maintaining the inpatient procedure code set. This manual is volume III of the ICD-10-CM manual.
* The *International Classification of Diseases, Tenth Revision, Clinical Modification (ICD-10-CM)* manual is used by physicians and other health-care providers to classify and code all diagnoses, symptoms, and procedures recorded in conjunction with hospital care in the United States. It is published by the WHO and uses unique alphanumeric codes to identify health-related conditions, diseases, signs and symptoms, and injuries and their causes. The National Center for Health Statistics (NCHS) is respon-sible for maintaining the manual, which includes more than 68,000 codes. The WHO released ICD-11-CM in June 2018; it will not go into effect until January 1, 2022.
* Health-care providers use this coding system in **outpa-tient diagnostic care.**
  * The manual is organized in the following way:
    * Introduction
    * Conversion table (developed by the NCHS to facilitate data retrieval as new codes are added to ICD-10-CM)
    * Official ICD-10-CM conventions and guidelines
    * Alphabetical index to diseases
    * Neoplasm table
    * Table of drugs and chemicals
    * Index of external causes
    * Tabular list of diseases
    * Appendixes

- Use the alphabetical index to begin your search for a code. It includes the following:
  - Diseases and injuries
  - External causes of injuries
  - Neoplasm table
  - Drugs and chemicals table
- The tabular listing is divided into 22 chapters and code ranges that are based on body system (site or condition).
  - This section is the final step for code confirmation.
- The chapters within the tabular listing are the following:
  - 1: Certain Infectious and Parasitic Diseases (A00-B99)
  - 2: Neoplasms (C00-D49)
  - 3: Diseases of the Blood and Blood Forming Organs and Certain Disorders Involving the Immune Mechanism (D50-D89)
  - 4: Endocrine, Nutritional, and Metabolic Diseases (E00-E89)
  - 5: Mental, Behavioral, and Neurodevelopmental Disorders (F01-F99)
  - 6: Diseases of the Nervous System (G00-G99)
  - 7: Diseases of the Eye and Adnexa (H00-H59)
  - 8: Diseases of the Ear and Mastoid Process (H60-H95)
  - 9: Diseases of the Circulatory System (I00-I99)
  - 10: Diseases of the Respiratory System (J00-J99)
  - 11: Diseases of the Digestive System (K00-K95)
  - 12: Diseases of the Skin and Subcutaneous Tissue (L00-L99)
  - 13: Diseases of the Musculoskeletal System and Connective Tissue (M00-M99)
  - 14: Diseases of the Genitourinary System (N00-N99)
  - 15: Pregnancy, Childbirth, and the Puerperium (O00-O9A)
  - 16: Certain Conditions Originating in the Perinatal Period (P00-P96)
  - 17: Congenital Malformations, Deformations and Chromosomal Abnormalities (Q00-Q99)
  - 18: Symptoms, Signs, and Abnormal Clinical and Laboratory Findings (R00-R99)

- 19: Injury and Poisoning and Certain Other Consequences of External Causes (S00-T98)
- 20: External Causes of an Injury or Health Condition (V00-Y99)
- 21: Factors Influencing Health Status and Contact with Health Services (Z00-Z99); may be assigned to further explain reason for presenting for service (includes transfer between facilities)
- 22: Codes for Special Purposes (U00-U85); these codes capture special circumstances such as new diseases of uncertain etiology or emergency use codes (U00-U85). Examples: U07.0 Vaping Related Disorder; U07.1 COVID-19

ICD Categories, Subcategories, and Valid Codes

- The 1st character is a letter, followed by letters/numbers.
- The 1st 3 digits are the category.
- Each level of subdivision after a 3-digit category represents a subcategory.
- The final level of subdivision is a valid code; valid codes may be 3, 4, 5, 6, or 7 characters in length.
- An "X" is used as a placeholder to allow for future expansion.

Examination Hint

The 1st letter of a diagnosis code refers to its chapter location. For instance, a code beginning with the letter "N" means it is from the genitourinary system chapter. The examination may have questions asking you to determine whether the code correctly matches its definition.

Example: For N48.1, a correct match would be "Balanitis." An incorrect match would be "Cellulitis of left finger."

Notable Coding Conventions

Punctuation marks

( ) Parentheses: Enclose supplementary words; nonessential modifiers

[ ] Brackets: Enclose synonyms or explanatory phrases

: Colon: Seen after a term that needs modifiers

Abbreviations

NEC (not elsewhere classified): Specified code not available

NOS (not otherwise specified): Unspecified

Instructional notes

Includes: Seen after category. It defines or gives examples.

Excludes: This term is used when 2 conditions cannot occur together or when the excluded condition is not part of the condition represented by the code.

See and See Also: These indicate that another term should be referenced within the alphabetic index.

Code Also: Two codes may be required.

Code 1st: Sequence the underlying condition 1st, followed by manifestation (signs and symptoms).

Italicized type: Not to be used as a 1st listed diagnosis. It is chiefly responsible for the service provided.

Key words using green type: The color helps the coder quickly identify the key terms and correct code.

ICD Terminology

Late effects: The residual condition produced after the acute phase of injury or illness has terminated. This has no time limit and requires 2 codes.

Placeholder: X character. This is used within certain codes to allow for future expansion. It may be used as a 5th character placeholder for certain 6-character codes and used as a 6th character placeholder for a code requiring 7 characters.

Primary diagnosis code: This is the chief (most significant) condition for which services or procedures were provided in an outpatient setting.

Principal diagnosis code: Applies only to inpatient settings. After study, it is the condition responsible for a patient's admission to the hospital.

YOUR NOTES

_____

_____

_____

_____

_____

_____

_____

Billing and Fee Collection

Cycle Billing

* This system was developed to bill a set of patients at the same time each month according to the 1st letter of their last name (e.g., patients with last name beginning with A through F are billed the 10th of each month) or some other sorting method.
* Rationale
  * Billing workload is reduced by spreading the task throughout the month (less time consuming).
  * This ensures cash flow throughout the month (payments receipt).

Balance Billing

* The patient is billed for the difference between the charge and the insurance payment.

• This is done if the provider is not participating with the patient's insurance plan.

Types of Payment

• At time of service
• Bill with credit extension
• Insurance (3rd party)
• Outside collection agency

Credit Policy of Office

• Payment due dates
• Payment due at time of service
• Collection procedures, including use of agency
• Participating insurance companies and accepting assignment

Collection Agency

• This is billing of last resort.
• The agency keeps 40% to 60% of the collected amount.
• Do not send bills or discuss the account with the patient after submitting the account to an agency.

YOUR NOTES

_____

_____

_____

_____

_____

_____

_____

Sample Certification Test Questions

Now that you have studied this chapter, here are some sample certification test questions for you.

1. In the ICD-10-CM manual, the number of digits (characters) that could be required to provide the highest level of specificity is

    A. 4
    B. 5
    C. 6
    D. 7
    E. 8

2. The E&M codes located in the CPT manual begin with which of the following 2 digits?

    A. 00
    B. 90
    C. 99
    D. 97
    E. 96

3. The ICD-10-CM codes that refer to factors that may influence a patient's health status are

    A. E codes
    B. Z codes
    C. V codes
    D. A codes
    E. H codes

See the Appendix for the answers.

Remember to use Edge after you finish this chapter to test your knowledge. Directions for how to access Edge, as well as your access code, are located on the inside front cover of this text.

YOUR NOTES

_____

_____

_____

_____

_____

_____

_____

Chapter 7

Medical Office Communications

Often, the patient's first contact with a medical practice is the person speaking to the patient on the telephone. The manner in which the person speaks and listens creates the patient's first impression of the office. Therefore, good verbal communication skills and professionalism are required of medical assistants to help a medical office business thrive.

The chapter begins with verbal communication, which includes special circumstances that affect communication and telephone skills. The telephone skill area can be the weakest for new medical assistants entering the field. A discussion of concepts of professional behavior follows communication skills. Written communication is then introduced, beginning with the written telephone message. All other forms of written communication follow: mailing supplies, business letters, e-mail, instant messages, faxes, etc.

Information regarding medical office communication content within the various national certifying exams may be found in Chapter 1.

DAVIS edge.

Remember to use Edge after you finish this chapter to test your knowledge. Directions for how to access Edge, as well as your access code, are located on the inside front cover of this text.

Verbal Communication

For communication to take place, there must be a message, a sender of the message, and a receiver for the message. The communication must be effective and efficient. Verbal communication is affected by the emotions and attitudes of those involved, as well as their objectives, facial expressions, gestures, voice tones, postures, and, often, their sense of touch. The sender and receiver are influenced by their moral code and observations of one another. The interpersonal and nonverbal components of communication are covered in Chapter 4.

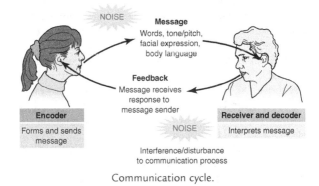

Communication cycle.

- Communication should strive to fulfill the "5 Cs." It should be
  - Clear
  - Cohesive
  - Complete
  - Concise
  - Courteous

Telephone Communication

Courtesy

- Using polite behavior (etiquette)
- Treating the caller with respect and tact
- Remaining calm at all times
- Answering an incoming call by identifying the office reached, followed by the office's telephone greeting policy
- Picking up a ringing telephone on the 1st ring and definitely by the 3rd ring

Inflection

- Changing one's pitch while speaking so as not to speak in a monotone

Pronunciation

- Saying words correctly to avoid any misunderstanding
- Avoiding the use of slang words, incorrect word contractions (e.g., whatcha, gotta), and words unfamiliar to the receiver of the message

Speed

- Speaking at a normal rate, not too slowly or hurriedly

Tone

- Controlling the overall sound quality of the voice to express a feeling, such as confidence, authority, compassion, or concern
- Using a pitch (highness or lowness) and timbre (resonance) of the voice that should be easy to listen to

Volume

- Keeping the voice at a normal level so the receiver does not strain to hear and also does not feel shouted at

Automated Voicemail Messaging

- This is a secure way to connect with groups of patients.
- Providers may communicate with patients regarding their health care
  - Leaving messages for patients on answering machines, cell phones
  - The amount of information disclosed should be limited

Telehealth Communication

- A means of communication that provides health-related services between patients and health-care providers. It allows this contact in order to provide care, advice, reminders, education, intervention, and monitoring. Telehealth helps patients and families find affordable and convenient health-care services. There are 4 types of telehealth.

- Live video conferencing: This is the most well-known. It is a live, 2-way, video-based communication between a patient and a health-care provider.
- Mobile health: Use of smart devices (phones, tablets, etc.) and health-based software. These apps encourage healthy lifestyles by monitoring such things as blood sugar levels of diabetics, etc.
- Remote patient monitoring: Most often used for seniors in senior living areas. A collection of a patient's health data from a patient or resident in one location is sent electronically to a health-care provider for monitoring or review.
- Asynchronous video: This is a documented and stored history that is forwarded outside of real time.

Communicating in Special Circumstances

Children

- Speak to children eye to eye (at their level).
- Always speak calmly and gently, and use short, simple sentences that are age appropriate.
- Always state the truth.
- Allow privacy from adults (especially adolescents) during assessment if desired.
- Encourage questions.

Geriatric Patients

- Ensure the patient's comfort, privacy, and safety in the examination room.
- Face the patient when speaking.
- Speak clearly and slowly. Do not shout.

Hearing Impaired Patients

- Communicate in a quiet environment.
- Speak clearly and slowly. Do not shout.

- Explain procedures carefully.
- Face the patient when speaking.
- Use a pen and paper for you and the patient to assist in communicating.

Non–English-Speaking Patients or Those With Limited Use of the Language

- Provide an interpreter if the patient has no friend or family to help interpret.
- Face the patient when speaking.
- Speak clearly using short, simple sentences.
- Use visual aids (demonstrations, pictures, and gestures).

Visually Impaired Patients

- Announce your presence.
- Offer your arm to guide patient through the facility.
- Explain all procedures thoroughly.
- Describe the surroundings to the patient.
- If necessary, leave the patient alone for only short amounts of time.
- Face the patient when speaking.

Related Terms and Definitions

Closed-ended questions: A question that requires a simple "yes," "no," or number response

Concise: Expressing a message clearly while using as few words as possible

Confidentiality: Keeping information private during a conversation or telephone call by being careful that the patient's name, symptom, or other information received is not overheard by those who do not need to know

Diction: Using the correct words pronounced carefully to be clear and effective

Effective use of silence: Giving the patient some time to think before responding; the patient may use the time to add helpful new information

Feedback: The response, either verbal or nonverbal, to a message

Jargon: The terminology commonly used by those in a given specialty field (Medical terminology should not be used when speaking to individuals not educated in the field.)

Open-ended questions: Questions that require more than "yes" or "no" responses (e.g., "Tell me about yourself.")

Paralanguage: The way a message is stated instead of the words in the message; refers to pitch, inflection, volume, speed of words spoken, and so forth

Paraphrasing or restating: Telling the messenger what you heard, in your own words

Reflecting: Repeating what is heard from the sender by using open-ended statements that the person must complete in response

Tactfulness: Choosing words carefully so as not to offend or upset someone receiving information from you

---

YOUR NOTES

_____

_____

_____

_____

_____

_____

Professionalism

Professional behavior produces a good work ethic and demonstrates the traits needed to perform well in a profession. You must show evidence of a businesslike manner, an appropriate appearance, and good hygiene. Standards of professionalism are set by organizations such as the American Medical Technologists (AMT), the American Association of Medical Assistants (AAMA), the National Center for Competency Testing (NCCT), and the American Medical Certification Association (AMCA). The following are important professional traits:

Coordination: The ability to plan and organize tasks to be accomplished by prioritizing within a time frame.

Critical thinking: The ability to evaluate situations and then take action based on the conclusions.

Determination: The willpower to overcome obstacles to complete the task at hand.

Diplomacy: The ability to communicate tactfully in a professional and courteous manner.

Discretion: The avoidance of commenting negatively about another medical office professional when speaking to patients. Discretion also includes not giving advice to patients unless specifically directed by the health-care provider to do so.

Integrity: This is the quality of being trustworthy and honest with physicians, employees, and patients. It includes the following: treating each patient with dignity and kindness; working within the law and in an ethical manner; completing all tasks before leaving at the end of the workday; and admitting your mistakes, thus ensuring high-quality care and lowering the chance for litigation.

Self-confidence: A belief in oneself and one's abilities. This is demonstrated by taking the initiative when working as a team member and is seen by the level of comfort patients and physicians have in the medical employee.

Understanding: The retention of knowledge and correct use of information. Expanding a knowledge base through continued education and comprehension increases understanding.

Written Communication

Any form of written communication to patients, coworkers, physicians, and all others speaks to the receiver about the professionalism of the entire medical facility. The receiver judges, by the sender's choice of words, conciseness, grammar, and spelling, whether the message was sent by a well-organized and competent facility or not. Medical and general dictionaries are essential tools for writing. Written correspondence serves as a legal record, so documents must be accurate and clear in their meaning.

Telephone Message Essentials

- Name of the person for whom the call was intended
- Date and time of the call
- Name of the individual calling
- Caller's cell phone number, work phone number, home phone number; hours during which to use each number; also the name and phone number of a pharmacy, if needed
- Detailed reason for the call
- Action that is required (e.g., call back, prescription refill)
- Initials of the person taking the message

Texting

- This form of communication is used when it is most appropriate to send a message from 1 cell phone to another. Most often, an office will text reminders to patients of upcoming office visits, request confirmation, and may give directions.

Business Letter Essentials

- Most business letters should be less than 1 page in length.
- The letter should be "you" oriented.
- It should be carefully organized.
- A draft of the letter should be written 1st; this allows an opportunity to reorganize and make corrections before finalization.

Paper

- **Bond**
  - Felt side and wire side; a watermark on the felt side is seen correctly when held up to the light
    - Watermark: An impression or design signifying high-quality paper
  - 25% or higher in cotton fiber content
- **Weight**
  - 20 to 24 lb (the higher the number, the heavier the paper)
  - 500 sheets per ream (10 reams to a case)
- **Size**
  - **Standard:** 8.5 × 11 inches (general business and professional correspondence)
  - **Monarch (executive):** 7.25 × 10.5 inches (office memorandum)
  - **Baronial:** 5.5 × 8.5 inches (½ of standard paper sheet); used for very short letters or memoranda

Envelopes

- Matching bond and color of letterhead paper
- Preprinted with office name and address in upper-left corner
- Commonly with a transparent address window used to view the recipient's mailing information printed on invoices and patient statements
- **Number 10:** For standard paper; most common "business" size
- **Number 6¾:** For baronial paper

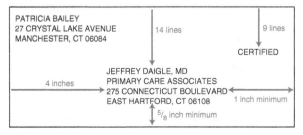

#10 envelope: Spacing, lettering, capitalization, punctuation, notations.

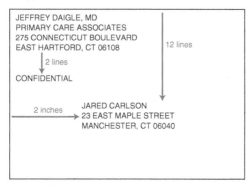

#6¾ envelope: Spacing, lettering, capitalization, punctuation, notations.

Parts of the Business Letter

The standard business letter contains 4 main parts:

- **Heading:** Letterhead and dateline
- **Opening:** Inside address, salutation, and attention line if required
- **Body:** Subject line if necessary, message
- **Closing:** Complimentary closing, typed signature, reference initials, and special notations (e.g., enclosures, copies to)

Format

- The letter should be single spaced.
- **Dateline:** Typed on line 15 if using no letterhead or 2 to 3 lines below the letterhead. Type the full name of the month, the day, and the full year (e.g., September 9, 2014).
- **Inside address:** This is typed on the 4th line below the dateline.
- **Salutation:** Typed on the 2nd line below the inside address. A colon follows the salutation. If a subject line is used, then the salutation will be typed on the 2nd line below the subject line.

- **Subject line:** Typed on the 2nd line below the inside address. It can begin at the left margin, indented 5 spaces, or it is centered.
- **Body of letter:** Begin typing on the 2nd line below the salutation or subject line.
- **Complimentary closing:** This is typed on the 2nd line below the last line of the letter body.
  - Formal style: "Respectfully yours" or "Respectfully"
  - General style: "Very truly yours" or "Truly yours"; or "Sincerely" or "Sincerely yours"
  - Informal style (when using 1st names): "Regards" or "Best wishes"
- **Keyed signature:** This is typed on the 4th line below the complimentary closing.
- **Reference initials:** Typed at the left margin, on the 2nd line below the keyed signature. A slash or colon is used to separate the composer from the typist; use uppercase for the composer and lowercase for the typist.
- **Enclosure notation:** If needed, type directly below the reference initials.
- **Copy notation:** If needed, type directly below the previously typed line.
- **Postscripts:** If needed, type on the 2nd line below the previously typed line.
- **Continuation page**
  - Begins 1 inch (line 7) from the top of the page
  - Required heading information for the 1st typed line:
    - Name of addressee
    - Page number
    - Date
  - The heading is used in the event that the pages of the document become separated.
  - The body of the letter begins on the 3rd line below the heading (10th line from the top).

Style

Full block: All typed lines begin at the left margin. It is the most efficient style, but it is less attractive on the page.

Modified block: All typed lines begin at the left margin, but the date line and complimentary closing are centered on the page.

Indented modified block: Each new paragraph begins with an indented line (5 spaces) by using the tab key.

Simplified: All typed lines begin at the left margin, and the salutation and complimentary closing are omitted. The subject line is typed in capital letters on the 3rd line below the inside address.

Memoranda (Interoffice Correspondence)

- Begin typing 2 inches (line 13) from the top of the page.
- The heading includes the following: date, to, from, and subject.

Heading Example #1

TO	All Staff
FROM	Kristen Correll, Office Manager
DATE	October 30, 2021
SUBJECT	Summer Staffing Schedule
	I will soon be planning for office staff coverage this upcoming summer season. If you know your summer vacation plans, please submit them at the next scheduled staff meeting on November 12 at 8:30 a.m.

Memorandum heading #1.

Heading Example #2

MEMO TO:	Clinical Supervisor, Claire Lorraine Administrative Supervisor, JoAnn Carlson
FROM:	Jeffrey Daigle, Office Manager
DATE:	September 29, 2021
SUBJECT:	Office Inventory

The new practice when receiving supplies (office and clinical) from vendors will be as follows:
1. Each box must be clearly marked with the date of receipt.
2. Each box must be numbered (1, 2, 3, etc.)
3. Begin using the highest numbered box. The last box opened will be #1.
4. Orders need not be made until the last box is opened for use.

Memorandum heading #2.

Editing and Proofreading

- These steps are performed when the 1st draft of a letter is completed.
- Editing is done by checking for clarity, flow of the letter, factual accuracy, conciseness, and correct letter style.
- Proofreading involves checking a document for any errors in grammar, spelling, and format.
- A good practice is to read the document from top to bottom for flow and clarity and then read it from bottom to top for spelling.
- Use the following tools for editing and proofreading: dictionary, medical dictionary, thesaurus, *Physicians' Desk Reference* (PDR), computer spell-checker (do not rely on this alone), and English grammar manual.
- When complete, have someone else proofread the letter as well.

?	is this correct?	⌐	move down
/	delete or change	¬	move up
^	insert a character	⌒	close up space
≡	set in capital letter(s)	sp	spell out
[	move to the left	⊙	insert period
]	move to the right	¶	new paragraph
#	insert a space	\ or ℘	delete
/ or lc	use lowercase	⋏	insert comma

Proofreading marks.

Computer Communications

E-mail

E-mails are written communications transmitted electronically from 1 computer user to 1 or more recipients.

- Office personnel communicating by e-mail must use the same professional tone as they use in a business letter.
- As with conventional letters, there are many formats and templates for e-mail letters.

- Use a variation of a simplified letter style, without the inside address and subject line.
- If the message is patient related, it must remain confidential. A printed copy of the e-mail is placed in the patient's chart.
- An e-mail may be used to remind patients of scheduled appointments.
- E-mails are often used in place of interoffice memoranda (use the office format).
- E-mails do not need a letterhead, inside address, or dateline.
- The message must use proper grammar and punctuation in the body of the letter. Common "texting" acronyms should never be used.
- Be sure to edit and proofread all e-mail messages before sending them.
- Business contact information should be added following the body of the message, including the business name, telephone number, fax number, and other contact information. Usually, an e-mail signature block has already been created to insert here.

Instant Messaging

Instant messaging is a type of online chatting. It uses real-time transmission over the Internet.

- The sender sets up a specific list of contacts, which may include professional contacts outside the medical office and patients, to receive this form of communication.
- It is often used to communicate with other personnel within the office.
- It should be checked frequently throughout office hours for risk management. Risk management involves the identifying, assessing, and controlling actions to minimize and prevent loss to a business because of legal liability.

Patient Portal

- It gives patients 24-hour access to their PHI (personal health information).
- This is a secure online website.

- Mainly used to:
  - Retrieve laboratory results
  - Send messages to their health-care provider and/or ask a question
  - Update patient profiles and insurance providers
- Some portals allow patients to schedule office visits and/or pay bills directly through the system.

Zoom

- This is a means of video communication with an easy, reliable cloud platform for video and audio conferencing, collaboration, and chatting.
- It gives the ability to host calls with others.
- Chat rooms can accommodate up to 500 attendees.

Skype

- This means of communication for business has many of the same features as Zoom; however, for business it excels as an office communications solution.
- It connects easily and quickly using instant messaging, screen and document sharing, and informed audio/video calls.

YOUR NOTES

_____

_____

_____

_____

_____

_____

_____

Sample Certification Test Questions

Now that you have studied this chapter, here are some sample certification test questions for you.

1. General and medical dictionaries are

- A. Not necessary if you have a word-processing spell-checker in your computer
- B. Necessary only if you have trouble with spelling
- C. Essential tools for every medical office
- D. Books to study and learn from while you are in school
- E. A and D

2. Answering the office telephone by saying only "Hello"

- A. Saves time
- B. Makes a caller feel rushed
- C. Is okay if you are in a hurry
- D. Makes callers think they have the wrong number
- E. None of the above

3. Which of the following dates is written correctly for inclusion in the heading of a letter?

- A. October 18th, 2021
- B. 10/18/21
- C. 10/18/2021
- D. October 18, '21
- E. October 18, 2021

See the Appendix for the answers.

Remember to use Edge after you finish this chapter to test your knowledge. Directions for how to access Edge, as well as your access code, are located on the inside front cover of this text.

YOUR NOTES

_____

_____

_____

_____

_____

_____

_____

Part 3

Clinical

Chapter 8
Clinical Skills

This chapter emphasizes the clinical knowledge and skills that you must know when working with providers and patients. You will be responsible for several components that assist providers with physical examinations. These components include gathering patient information (e.g., history and vital statistics). They also include equipment sanitization, disinfection, and sterilization; medical and surgical asepsis; patient positioning and gowning; examination equipment and supply maintenance; physical therapies; and recognizing emergencies and first-aid application. Also covered in this chapter are common abbreviations; physical examination information for adults, infants, and toddlers; and nutrition. Your mastery of all these components helps ensure a smooth office operation.

Information regarding clinical content within the various national certifying exams may be found in Chapter 1.

Remember to use Edge after you finish this chapter to test your knowledge. Directions on how to access Edge, as well as your access code, are found on the inside front cover of this text.

Common Medical Documentation Abbreviations

Abbreviation	Meaning
ABC	Airway, breathing, circulation
AD	Right ear (auris dexter)
AK	Above the knee
ALL	Allergy
ama	Against medical advice
ANS	Autonomic nervous system
A&P	Anterior and posterior; auscultation and percussion
AS	Left ear (auris sinister)
AU	Both ears together (aures unitas)
A&W	Alive and well
BK	Below the knee
BM	Bowel movement
BP, B/P	Blood pressure
BPM	Beats per minute
BRAT	Bananas, rice, applesauce, and toast (diet helps control diarrhea)
C	Celsius
CA	Cancer
CC or cc	Chief complaint
CNS	Central nervous system
C/O	Complains of
CXR	Chest x-ray
DASH	Fresh fruits, vegetables, no alcohol, low salt, high fiber (diet helps lower BP)

Abbreviation	Meaning
D&C	Dilation and curettage
DNR	Do not resuscitate
Dx	Diagnosis
EMS	Emergency medical services
ENT	Ears, nose, throat
Eq	Equivalent
ER	Emergency room
F	Fahrenheit
FH	Family history
f/u	Follow up
FUO	Fever of undetermined origin
FYI	For your information
GI	Gastrointestinal
HBP	High blood pressure
HEENT	Head, ears, eyes, nose, throat
H&P	History and physical
HPI	History of present illness
HR	Heart rate
HRT	Hormone replacement therapy
Hx	History
ICU	Intensive care unit
I&D	Incision and drainage
L&A	Light and accommodation
LBP	Low blood pressure
LMP	Last menstrual period

Continued

Abbreviation	Meaning
L&W	Living and well
MA	Mental age
N/O	No complaints
OD	Right eye (oculus dexter)
OS	Left eye (oculus sinister)
OU	Each eye (oculus uterque)
PE, Ex	Physical examination
PERRLA	Pupils equal, round, reactive to light and accommodation
PH	Past history
PNS	Peripheral nervous system
PT	Physical therapy
Px	Prognosis
REM	Rapid eye movement
ROM	Range of motion
ROS	Review of systems
SH	Social history
SIDS	Sudden infant death syndrome
SOB	Shortness of breath
Sx	Symptoms
TIA	Transient ischemic attack
TPR	Temperature, pulse, respiration
Tx	Treatment
UTI	Urinary tract infection
VS	Vital signs
WNL	Within normal limits

Asepsis

Asepsis is the state of being free from pathogens (bacteria, viruses, fungi, parasites). Aseptic technique is the use of measures that prevent contact with disease-causing contaminants. Elimination of infection is the general goal of asepsis. There are 2 types of asepsis practiced in the medical field: medical asepsis and surgical asepsis.

Medical Asepsis

The goals of medical asepsis are maintaining cleanliness and preventing the spread of all pathogenic microorganisms through good hygienic practice. Medical asepsis is used for the following:

- Dermal patch application
- Oral, rectal, or tympanic temperature measurement
- Venipuncture
  - Uses routine antiseptic hand washing, disposable nonsterile gloves, fast-acting antiseptic (alcohol), and a thoroughly cleaned skin puncture site
- Cerumen removal
- Proctoscopy
- Blood pressure (BP) measurement
- Eye irrigation or instillation

Hand Washing

Correct hand washing is the most important single method of asepsis.

Medical Aseptis Hand Washing

- Keep the hands lower than the forearms (water flows into the sink instead of back onto the arms).
- With the water running, dry the hands with clean, dry paper towels, and then turn off the faucets using a clean, dry paper towel.

Surgical Asepsis Hand Washing

- Use a sterile scrub brush.
- Wash the hands and forearms.
- Hold the hands higher than the elbows (water cannot flow from the arms onto the washed areas).
- Use **sterile towels** instead of paper towels.

Surgical Asepsis

The goal of surgical asepsis is the exclusion of *all* microorganisms. This form of asepsis is used during most or all sterile invasive procedures, including venipuncture and parenteral administration (e.g., Mantoux tuberculin skin test and phlebotomy). It is also used when gloving, setting up, and maintaining a sterile tray for the following:

- Venipuncture and parenteral administration
- Suture removal
- Dressing change
- Urinary catheter insertion
- Minor laceration closure
- Sterile solution pouring
- Local infection incision and drainage (I&D)
- Culture collection

Guidelines for Surgical Asepsis

- A 1-inch border around the sterile field is considered contaminated.
- Hold sterile items above the waist; below the waist is considered contaminated.
- Always face the sterile field, and never reach over the field.
- Place items in the center of the field.
- If you must leave the field, place a sterile towel over the field.
- Never cough or sneeze over a sterile field.
- If a sterile object comes in contact with an unsterile item, it is considered contaminated and cannot be used.

- If in doubt about the sterility of an item, **DO NOT USE.**
- If the sterile field has been broken, start all over with setup.
- For venipuncture and parenteral administration:
  - You must use and maintain sterile equipment for the invasive procedure.
  - Any introduction of a sterile item into a patient must always be performed with a no-touch technique.
- Skin should not be touched in the area of insertion after skin antiseptic is used.
- The sterile devices must not touch nonsterile surfaces.

Sanitization, Disinfection, and Sterilization

Antiseptics

- Antiseptics are used to cleanse infective agents from human skin and wounds.
- Applicators include alcohol wipes, sponges, and cotton tips.
- Prepare the patient's skin by using an outward circular motion from an incision site for 2 to 5 minutes.

Sanitization

- The cleaning (scrubbing process) of debris, blood, and pathogenic microorganisms from instruments, equipment, and the examining room. Use disinfectant or detergent solution (with low suds and neutral pH) to soak the instruments; then drain the sink and use hot, soapy water and scrub with a nonmetal scrub brush.
- For some instruments, this is the first step before disinfection and sterilization.

Disinfection

- This refers to the reduction of the number of pathogenic microorganisms on objects or in materials so that they pose no threat of disease.

- It involves the use of chemicals on instruments, equipment, and countertops. Chemicals include glutaraldehyde (Cidex), chemical germicides, and household bleach (sodium hypochlorite).

Sterilization

- This method destroys all microorganisms by dry heat, steam heat, chemicals, or gases.
  - **Gases** for large equipment (e.g., beds); used in hospitals
  - **Dry heat** for instruments prone to corrosion
  - **Chemicals** for heat-sensitive equipment
  - **Steam heat** (autoclave) for heat- and moisture-stable instruments and equipment
- Steam heat sterilization is the most common method in medical offices. The procedure is as follows:
  - Operate with distilled water.
  - Wrap instruments (hinged instruments are wrapped in the open position).
  - Steam temperature must be 250°F to 254°F.
  - For effective sterilization, sterilize for 20 to 40 minutes.
  - Begin timing when indicators show the recommended temperature and pressure.
  - The maximum shelf life for a sterile pack is 30 days.

Gathering Patient Information

History

Medical practices keep a history of each patient's medical treatment. The history must be thorough to provide a foundation for all current and future care of the patient by the practice. The following areas are covered in a patient's history:

- Presenting problem: Reason for the visit (chief complaint [CC])
- Signs (objective findings): Observed, test results, examination results

- Symptoms (subjective findings): Patient provides information (e.g., pain scale 1 to 10). Children are given the opportunity to express symptoms in their own words.
- Past and present diseases
- Medical problems
- Medications, including any over-the-counter (OTC) medications
- Pregnancies and births
  - Example: Three children, 1 set of twins, 2 spontaneous abortions, and 1 abortion are documented as **G** 5 = **number of pregnancies, P** 3 = **number of live births, Ab** 1 = **number of abortions.**
- Allergies and other peculiarities (anatomical abnormalities)
- Past surgeries and injuries
- Social history: Alcohol, drugs, and sexual orientation
- Mental health: Past and present
- Family history: Causes of death, diseases

Vital Statistics

The term means the vital signs plus mensuration (height and weight). The information received from all these measurements is useful in assessing the present health of the patient and the patient's progress, diagnoses, and variations from normal ranges of individuals, as well as for tracking the patient's illnesses.

Vital Signs

Providers measure vital signs to determine how well the patient's body is functioning. Vital signs include temperature, pulse, respiration, and BP.

Temperature

Under healthy conditions, the temperature of a person averages 98.6° Fahrenheit (F) or 37° Celsius (C). Body temperature varies slightly with individuals. The average range in healthy adults is 97°F to 99°F (36.1°C to 37.2°C). A core temperature over 100.4°F (38°C) is defined as a fever by an illness or infection.

Pyrexia: The medical term for fever

Febrile: Describes a patient with fever

- **Low body temperature causes:**
  - Blood loss
  - Fainting
  - Dehydration
  - Fasting
  - Central nervous system injury

Average Body Temperature		
Anatomical Site	°F (Fahrenheit) Average	°C (Celsius) Average
Oral: under tongue in mouth	98.6	36.8
Rectal (R): rectum used before age of 3 Most accurate, gold standard	100 (R)	37.8 (R)
Axillary (A): in armpit area (least accurate)	97.6 (A)	36.4 (A)
Tympanic (T): eardrum (quick and easy) **Adults:** Pull ear up and back **Children:** Pull ear down and back	100 (T)	37.8 (T)
Digital: not 100% accurate, general sense of true temperature	98.6	36.8
Laser infrared: noncontact, accuracy within ± 0.6°F (±0.3°C)	98.6	36.8

Pulse

A person's pulse is an indicator of heart and blood vessel function. It is an indirect measure of cardiac output. A healthy pulse has a regular rhythm and rate, and it is easily palpated.

- Measure by applying gentle pressure to the artery against bone at the site. Do not use your thumb to measure—it has a pulse.

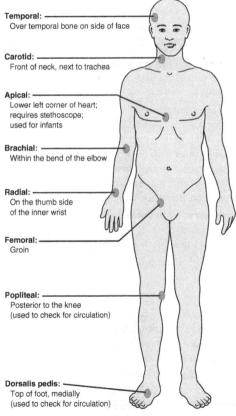

Temporal:
Over temporal bone on side of face

Carotid:
Front of neck, next to trachea

Apical:
Lower left corner of heart; requires stethoscope; used for infants

Brachial:
Within the bend of the elbow

Radial:
On the thumb side of the inner wrist

Femoral:
Groin

Popliteal:
Posterior to the knee (used to check for circulation)

Dorsalis pedis:
Top of foot, medially (used to check for circulation)

Anatomical pulse sites.

- Pulse-taking on infants requires the use of a stethoscope.
- Rate is equal to the number of heartbeats felt in a minute (bpm).
- Rhythm is the regular, recurrent expansion and contraction of an artery.
- Volume is strength, the force of the pulse.
- The adult rate is 60 to 100 bpm; the rate in children is 70 to 120 bpm.
- Common pulse sites are shown in the illustration.

Arrhythmia: Irregular beat

Bradycardia: Slow, regular beat (less than 60 bpm)

Bruit: Sound made by blockage in the carotid artery

Extrasystole: An extra (beat) heart contraction, which interrupts the normal, regular rhythm of the heart

Pulse oximetry: A simple, painless, noninvasive test. A small clip-on device gently attaches to a part of the body that is translucent enough to let light pass through (e.g., earlobe, fingertip, toe) and measures the percent of oxygenated hemoglobin (Hgb); 95% or higher is normal; it is used to assess and monitor pulmonary function of patients with pneumonia, bronchitis, emphysema, and asthma, as well as those handling increased activity levels.

Pulse pressure: Difference between systolic and diastolic reading. It gives tone of arterial walls; higher than 50 or lower than 30 mm Hg is abnormal.

Tachycardia: Rapid, regular beat (usually greater than 90 bpm)

Respiration

Respiration refers to the act of breathing (inspiration or inhalation and exhalation). Respiration works with the heart and circulation to remove waste products and provide nourishment to the body's cells.

- The adult rate is 12 to 20 breaths per minute (count chest risings); the rate in children is 18 to 30 breaths per minute.
- The ratio of respirations to pulse rate is 1 breath to 4 pulse beats (1:4): evenly spaced, of moderate depth, and quiet.

Dyspnea: Difficult or painful breathing

Eupnea: Normal breathing

Exhalation: The lungs deflate, and the diaphragm rises to assist the lungs

Hyperpnea: Rapid, deep breathing

Inspiration (inhalation): The lungs fill, and the diaphragm moves down to allow expansion

Tachypnea: Rapid breathing

Blood Pressure: The Arterial Pressure Measurement

The measurement of BP is a means of assessing the health of the patient's heart and blood vessels.

- BP measures the force of blood against the artery walls.
- It is measured in millimeters of mercury (mm Hg).
- A common site is the brachial artery located at the inside elbow of the arm.
- The left arm gives a slightly higher reading.
- Do not press your thumb on the stethoscope bell. Your thumb has a pulse.
- BP rises with age because of the loss of elasticity in blood vessels.
- The first sound is systolic.
- The last sound is diastolic.

Systolic: The pressure produced on the artery vessel as the left ventricle contracts and sends blood into arteries. Normal adult systolic BP is less than 120 mm Hg.

Diastolic: The relaxation phase of the heart as the left ventricle refills with blood. Normal adult diastolic BP is less than 80 mm Hg.

Korotkoff's sounds: These are the sounds between the 1st and last sounds.

Sphygmomanometer: This device is used to measure BP. The parts of the sphygmomanometer are as follows:

- **Dial:** This registers pressure (mm Hg).
- **Cuff:** This regulates the flow of blood through blood vessels.

- **Pressure bulb:** This is used to pump air into the cuff. Inflate the cuff 20 mm Hg above the point at which the radial pulse disappears.
- **Control valve:** This controls the release of air from the cuff.

Vision Testing

Testing the patient's vision may be done as part of a routine physical examination. The Snellen chart (random characters arranged in rows of the same size in each row) is used most often.

- The chart is made up of rows of letters. From top to bottom, the letters in each row decrease in size.
- The patient stands 20 feet (6 m) from the chart. Each eye is tested separately; then both eyes are tested together.
- A measurement of 20/30 means that the smallest line an eye, with less visual acuity, sees at 20 feet is seen by a normal eye at 30 feet.
- A measurement of 20/40-1 means that the smallest line an eye, with less visual acuity, sees at 20 feet is seen by a normal eye at 40 feet minus 1 letter in the line.

Color Blindness Testing

- In most instances, the reader needs to identify various characters on a set of 24 color test plates from the PseudoIsochromatic Plate Ishihara Color Vision Test book.
- Green and red color blindness is the most common type of abnormal color perception.
- Color blindness occurs in more male than female patients.

Common Examination Terminology

Auscultation: This means listening to body sounds with a stethoscope.

Inspection: This is a visual examination of the patient (size, shape, symmetry, abnormalities, and skin color and condition).

Manipulation: Body parts are moved to assess range of motion.

Palpation: Touching the skin surface and using some pressure to feel underlying organs to assess texture, temperature, movement, and shape.

Percussion: Listening to body sounds by tapping body areas to assess resonance of appropriate organs and body cavities (e.g., lungs).

Romberg balance test: To assess muscle abnormalities. The patient stands with feet together, eyes closed.

Newborn, Infant, and Toddler Examination

- Length and weight are taken and plotted on a growth chart.
- Immunizations are administered according to the immunization schedule.
- Denver II Developmental Screening Test
  - This test screens gross and fine motor skills, personal skills, and development.
  - It is administered periodically between 1 month and 6 years of age.

Newborns

- Newborns are assessed for an **Apgar score** 1 and 5 minutes after birth.
  - The Apgar score measures 5 signs: appearance (color), pulse, grimace (reflex to stimuli), activity (muscle tone), and respiration.
  - Each sign is scored with a 0, 1, or 2 and is totaled.
  - Newborns scoring lower than 7 need medical attention.
- For BP, 60–96/30–62 mm Hg is the approximate range.
- 98.2°F (axillary) is the temperature average.
- They receive the 1st hepatitis B immunization.

Infants and Toddlers

- Infants are up to 1 year old.
- Toddlers are from 1 up to 3 years old.
- Head circumference measurement is made just above the eyebrows and the top of the ears (widest measure); it is performed until 36 months of age.

- Infant pulse (apical) ranges from 100 to 160 bpm (use stethoscope, measure for 1 full minute, and document as a number and "AP" [apical]).

Positioning and Gowning

Preparing the patient: Explain the examination (purpose and positioning) and ask the patient whether he or she needs assistance.

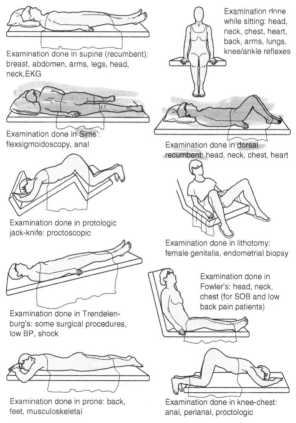

Examination done in supine (recumbent): breast, abdomen, arms, legs, head, neck, EKG

Examination done while sitting: head, neck, chest, heart, back, arms, lungs, knee/ankle reflexes

Examination done in Sims': flexsigmoidoscopy, anal

Examination done in dorsal recumbent: head, neck, chest, heart

Examination done in protologic jack-knife: proctoscopic

Examination done in lithotomy: female genitalia, endometrial biopsy

Examination done in Trendelenburg's: some surgical procedures, low BP, shock

Examination done in Fowler's: head, neck, chest (for SOB and low back pain patients)

Examination done in prone: back, feet, musculoskeletal

Examination done in knee-chest: anal, perianal, proctologic

Positioning and gowning.

Common Instruments for Physical Examination

Ishihara color number plate: Tests for color blindness

Nasal speculum: To check the structures of the nose in adults

Ophthalmoscope: To check the health of the eyes; "red reflex" indicates good health

Otoscope: To examine the inner structures of the ear

Penlight: To check pupil response to light; to check the nasal passages, tongue, and mouth

Percussion hammer: To check reflexes (neurological evaluation)

Pinwheel: To check touch sensation

Pupil tonometer: Tests for glaucoma

Snellen chart: Used most often to test vision

Sphygmomanometer: To check BP

Stethoscope: Used for auscultation

Tape measure: Compares measurements of limbs and the circumference of an infant's head

Thermometer: To check temperature

Tongue depressor and laryngeal mirror: To check the mouth and throat

YOUR NOTES

_____

_____

_____

_____

_____

_____

_____

Tuning fork: Used to assess hearing; size C most commonly used

Vaginal speculum: To check the structure of the vagina

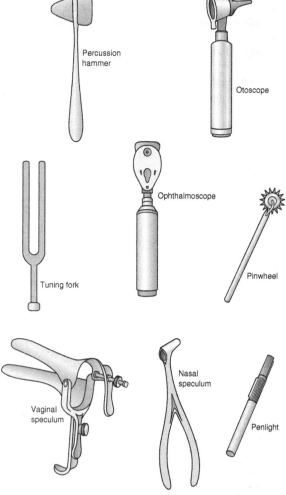

Common instruments for physical examination.

Special Equipment

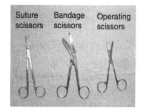

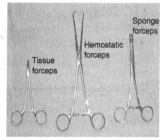

Instruments: Terms and Functions	
Function	**Instrument**
Cutting	Scissors and scalpel
Grasping or clamping	Hemostat, forceps, clamp, and needle holder
Probing or dilating	Speculum, scope, probe, retractor, and dilator
Vaporizing tissues	Laser
Sewing tissues	Suture (noun; material used to sew)

Nutrition

Nutrition is defined as the processes that occur because of nutrient intake and their utilization. Nutrition is the key to metabolism. Metabolism relies on nutrients that break down to produce energy.

Dietary Factors

Basal metabolic rate (BMR): This represents energy used while fasting or resting to maintain vital functions.

Metabolism: All the chemical reactions that occur within the cells of living organisms that allow growth, reproduction, energy production, and waste excretion. Metabolism has 2 categories: anabolism and catabolism.

- **Anabolism:** Uses energy to construct components of cells (proteins and nucleic acids)
- **Catabolism:** Breaks down organic matter and receives energy through cellular respiration (e.g., glycogen conversion to glucose)

Calorie: A unit of heat energy. It is the amount of oxygen (O_2) used.

Nutrients: Nutrients consist of carbohydrates, proteins, and fats. They are essential to supply energy (calories) from chemicals in food that the body cannot synthesize.

- **Carbohydrates**
  - For energy; classified by complexity
  - A simple sugar (i.e., white bread, rice, potatoes, pasta)
  - A complex plant food (i.e., most vegetable and fruit produce)
- **Proteins**
  - Build and repair body tissue
  - Composed of amino acids
- **Fats**
  - For energy and heat
  - Saturated: Animal fat
  - Unsaturated: Liquid at room temperature
  - Monounsaturated: Olives, avocados
  - Polyunsaturated: Nuts, seeds

Daily Nutrition	
Food Group	Daily Recommendation
Grains: Highest daily amount	At least 3 oz of "whole" grain
Vegetables	Variety: more dark green and orange
Fruits	Variety: fresh, frozen, canned, and dried; less juice

Daily Nutrition—cont'd

Food Group	Daily Recommendation
Dairy	Low-fat or no-fat
Meat and beans	Low-fat or lean meats, poultry, fish (bake, broil, grill), nuts, and beans
Oils: Lowest daily amount	Fish, nuts, and vegetables; less solid fat (butter or shortening); no trans fats

Vitamins

Vitamin	Function
A	Fat soluble, beta carotene, prevents night blindness
E	Fat soluble, anticoagulant
D	Fat soluble, for calcium absorption, lowers risk of rickets and osteomalacia
K	Fat soluble, for blood clotting, lowers risk of hemorrhage
C	Water soluble, lowers risk of scurvy, heals wounds, protects against infection
B complex	Water soluble, supports metabolism, promotes hemoglobin formation
Folic acid	Water soluble, for red blood cell production, liver health

Minerals

Mineral	Function
Calcium	Bone building, cardiac function, muscle contraction, blood coagulation
Chloride	Body pH and fluid balance

Continued

Minerals—cont'd	
Mineral	Function
Phosphorus	Metabolism of protein, calcium, and glucose
Sodium	Body pH balance, muscle contraction control; level regulated by kidneys
Potassium	Protein synthesis, pH balance, heartbeat regulation
Magnesium	Bone building, metabolism, enzyme activities
Zinc	Growth, healing, sense of taste, glucose tolerance
Iron	Hemoglobin component needed for O_2 transport through body

YOUR NOTES

_____

_____

_____

_____

_____

_____

_____

Physical Therapies

Thermotherapy

- The application of dry or moist heat for pain relief
- Lowers occurrences of muscle spasms and localized swelling
- Encourages tissue repair

- Encourages infected area drainage
- Types of thermotherapy:
  - **Diathermy**
    - Producing heat in body tissues by high-frequency currents
    - Used for arthritis, tendonitis
  - **Ultraviolet**
    - Controlled lamp exposure therapy (e.g., for rickets, psoriasis)
  - **Ultrasound**
    - Uses water-soluble gel and high-frequency sound waves
    - Most common use of diathermy
  - **Cryotherapy**
    - Application of dry or moist cold; used for:
      - Vasoconstriction
      - Involuntary muscle contraction
      - Decreasing blood supply to area
      - Numbing effect on nerve endings
      - Controlling bleeding or swelling
      - Pain

Massage

- Massage is used to lower pain and muscle tension.

Electric Muscle Stimulation

- Transcutaneous electric nerve stimulation (TENS) unit is used for orthopedics such as:
  - Arthritis
  - Back injury
  - Sports injury
- It is not for patients with cardiac disease or pacemakers because of electrical stimulation.

Traction

- Part of the body is pulled or stretched to:
  - Align bones or relieve vertebral bone compression
  - Reduce or relieve muscle spasms and shortenings

Mobility Devices

- Walkers: The top of the walker should be just below the waist, the same height as the top of the hip bone; elbows bend at 30° while using.
- Crutches: These should reach 1 to 1.5 inches below the armpits; handgrips are at the top of the hip line; the patient stands on the good leg and moves the crutches ahead of the good foot.

Crutch Walking Patterns

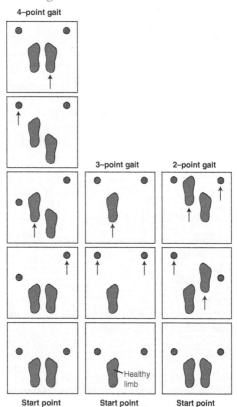

YOUR NOTES

_____

_____

_____

_____

_____

_____

Office Preparedness for Emergencies

A written plan should be in place, and personnel should have specific roles and responsibilities assigned to them in case of any office emergency. Because of personnel turnover and needed refreshing, a review of the plan should be done quarterly.

• Emergency exits and exit directions must be posted in every room.
• Emergency telephone numbers must be readily available (e.g., ambulance, hospital, poison control, etc.).

Medical Office Emergency Equipment

• Cardiac code cart
• IV supplies
• O_2 with mask delivery
• Cold packs
• Wound care kit
• Personal protective equipment (PPE)
• Childbirth or delivery kit
• AED (automated external defibrillator)

An AED is a crucial necessity that helps to restart the heart and assist in re-establishing an effective rhythm cycle.

Proper pad placement allows the electrical shock to travel through the victim's heart. For adults, the pad placement is as follows:

- One pad is placed on the anterior of the chest wall, above the right nipple and below the victim's clavicle.
- The second pad is placed on the left side of the chest wall below the breast area.

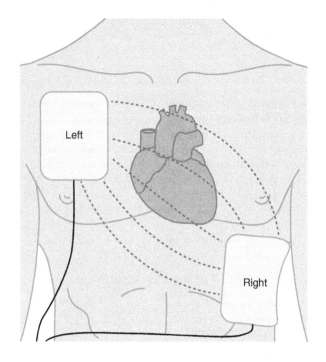

Medical Emergencies, First Aid, and Cardiopulmonary Resuscitation

A medical emergency is a situation in which a person's life is threatened as a result of injury or illness. Immediate help or first aid may be required to sustain life, prevent further injury, reduce pain, minimize the consequences of respiratory and cardiac emergencies, and increase early recovery chance until more advanced medical help arrives. Take the following sequence of actions when arriving at emergency scenes:

- Check the scene for safety.
  - Is it safe to go into the site? What happened? How many people are involved? Is anyone else available to help?
  - Can you treat victims at the site or remove them safely from it?
- Check for life-threatening conditions.
  - No signs of life (breathing, movement)
  - Unconsciousness
    - Convulsions
  - Respiratory distress
  - Severe bleeding
    - Deep wound
  - Chest or other severe pain
- Call 9-1-1.
  - This sends emergency medical services (EMS) to the scene as soon as possible.
- Check a second time for the following:
  - Level of consciousness (ask name and date)
    - Mental orientation
  - Vital signs
  - Skin color and moisture
    - Abnormal skin color
  - Palpate for pain
    - Bone fracture
    - Bleeding
- Care for the injured or ill person, but *if you are alone*, take these actions:
  - Call 9-1-1 first:
    - If someone is unconscious (adult, adolescent, child, or infant)
    - If you have witnessed the sudden collapse of an infant or child

- Care first (up to 2 minutes):
  - Any drowning person
  - An unwitnessed adolescent, child, or infant collapse and unconsciousness

The American Red Cross ABCs of Cardiopulmonary Resuscitation (CPR)

- **A**: Check **a**irway.
- **B**: Look, listen, and feel for **b**reathing.
- **C**: Check the carotid artery for **c**irculation (pulse).

The American Heart Association CABs of Cardiopulmonary Resuscitation (CPR)

- **C**: Assess **c**irculation, start **c**ompressions if no pulse
- **A**: Open **a**irway
- **B**: Give **b**reaths

First Aid

Burns

Type	Care
First degree: red, no blister	Immerse in cool water Apply sterile, cool, wet compress
Second degree: red, blistering	Immerse in cool water 1–2 hours Cover with dry, sterile dressing
Third degree: full skin thickness, may involve muscle tissue	Cover with thick, dry, sterile dressing or dressing soaked in sterile saline solution if available Do not pull off adhered clothing because of infection and dehydration risk
Chemical	If powdered agent, try to brush off; if not, rinse copiously, then cover with sterile dressing

Myocardial Infarction (MI)

Signs and Symptoms	Care
Chest pain, left arm pain, jaw pain, sweating, indigestion, rapid respirations, nausea, and vomiting	Activate EMS Get code cart and O_2 Check ABCs if needed Check vital signs Keep patient calm

Convulsions

Signs and Symptoms	Care
Jerking, spasmodic body movements, loss of consciousness	Activate EMS Protect head Maintain airway

Stroke: Cerebrovascular Accident (CVA)

Signs and Symptoms	Care
Slurred speech, confusion, paralysis to 1 side of body, unequal pupils	Activate EMS Maintain airway Check vital signs Keep patient calm

Bleeding

Type	Care
Bleeding from limb, head, or neck	Elevate injured part above heart if possible
All Types	
Severe bleeding	Apply direct pressure with sterile compress Add more compresses as needed—do not replace used compress; it disturbs clotting process If needed, use indirect pressure on pulse point between wound and heart to slow bleeding process Life-or-death situation: Last resort is tourniquet application; note time of application

Syncope

Signs and Symptoms	Care
Unconsciousness resulting from drop in BP or low level of O_2	Place in supine position with head lower than heart Maintain open airway Apply cool compress to forehead Loosen tight clothing

Shock

Signs and Symptoms	Care
Cool, pale, moist skin, low BP, weak or rapid pulse, agitation, restlessness, dyspnea, and weakness (may be caused by severe blood loss)	Activate EMS Maintain airway Place in Trendelenburg's position (if no head injury) Check vital signs Keep patient warm

- **Common types of shock**
  - **Anaphylactic:** Severe allergic reaction (low BP, edema, tachycardia, dyspnea)
  - **Cardiogenic:** Impaired cardiac function
  - **Hypovolemic** (hemorrhagic): Low blood volume
  - **Insulin:** Severe hypoglycemia
  - **Neurogenic:** Trauma to nervous system; fainting (blood vessels dilate, loss of tone, low BP and heart rate)
  - **Septic:** Infection that is spread by blood to all body systems
  - **Traumatic:** Loss of interstitial fluid (i.e., large burn areas)

Respiratory Distress

Type	Care
Asthma: Narrowing airways causing breathing difficulty or wheezing sound	Check ABCs (CABs) Have patient sit upright, if possible Assist with inhaler Monitor O_2 with pulse oximeter Keep patient calm

Type	Care
Hyperventilation: Leading to lower CO_2 level resulting in dizziness or unconsciousness	Place paper bag over patient's nose and mouth; have patient breathe slowly and calmly
Choking: Coughing audibly Choking: Clutching throat, unable to produce sound	Encourage patient to continue coughing Perform **Heimlich maneuver** ("bear hug" from behind, 1 hand covers balled fist below ribs and above navel, pull in with upward thrusts) to dislodge foreign object

Fractures

- **Types:** Refer to Chapter 3.
- **Care:** Immobilize with splint, elevate (if possible); apply ice packs; use slings for fractured clavicle or arms.

Poisoning

Type	Care
Inhaled, ingested, injected; chemical or natural	Activate EMS Call poison control for instructions Use personal protective equipment (PPE) Check ABCs Check vital signs

Diabetic Conditions

Type	Care
Insulin shock: Moist, pale skin; rapid heart rate; confusion	Give food containing sugar that will be rapidly absorbed (orange juice or glucose gel)
Diabetic coma: Dry, flushed skin; "fruity" breath; extreme thirst; confusion; rapid respiration	Activate EMS Provider must administer insulin

YOUR NOTES

_____

_____

_____

_____

_____

_____

Sample Certification Test Questions

Now that you have studied this chapter, here are some sample certification test questions for you.

1. When you are alone with an unresponsive teenage victim and no second rescuer is in the area, you should first:

   A. Wait for help to arrive.
   B. Open the victim's airway.
   C. Begin chest compressions.
   D. Call 9-1-1 to activate the EMS system.
   E. Position the victim on his or her back.

2. What does disinfection do to any surface?

   A. Removes blood
   B. Kills only pathogenic microorganisms
   C. Kills only the good and benign microorganisms
   D. Removes debris and blood
   E. Sterilizes it

3. Which of the following is true of vitamin D?

    A. It raises the rate of metabolism.

    B. It is water soluble.

    C. It is an anticoagulant.

    D. It enhances calcium absorption.

    E. It promotes blood clotting.

See the Appendix for the answers.

Remember to use Edge after you finish this chapter to test your knowledge. Directions for how to access Edge, as well as your access code, are located on the inside front cover of this text.

YOUR NOTES

_____

_____

_____

_____

_____

_____

_____

Chapter 9

Pharmacology

Pharmacology is the study of drugs and their origin, their nature and properties, and their effect on living organisms. For the most part, drugs are manufactured in laboratories, but many are obtained from animals, toxins, plants, and minerals. Medical assistants need to have a general knowledge of various types of drugs and their actions, uses, routes of administration, common side effects, and factors affecting their effects and elimination. In addition, you will be expected to know the following: common terminology used in pharmacology; common prescription abbreviations; the "7 rights" of drug administration; delivery systems; immunizations; and metric and household measurements and conversions. There may be examination questions on areas of related law and drug references. Finally, you should anticipate making simple dosage calculations.

To help you prepare, this chapter includes the abbreviations and terminology you may find embedded within test questions. You are expected to already know the meanings and apply them to the questions. The chapter also includes lists of the most commonly used drugs and their interactions and effects, along with summaries of all the other areas mentioned earlier.

Information regarding pharmacology content within the various national certifying exams may be found in Chapter 1.

Remember to use Edge after you finish this chapter to test your knowledge. Directions for how to access Edge, as well as your access code, are located on the inside front cover of this text.

Common Abbreviations

Abbreviation	Meaning
aa	Of each
a.c.	Before meals
AD	Right ear
ad lib	As desired
amt	Amount
aq	Water
AS	Left ear
AU	Both ears
bid	Twice a day
BSA	Body surface area
c	With
caps	Capsules
d/c, DC	Discontinue
disp	Dispense
dL	Deciliter
elix	Elixir
emul	Emulsion
et	And
fl	Fluid
hr	Hour
hs	Hour of sleep
K	Potassium
mcg	Microgram
n	Normal

Abbreviation	Meaning
NaCl	Sodium chloride
NPO	Nothing by mouth
OD	Right eye
Ophth	Instill in eyes
OS	Left eye
OTC	Over the counter
otic	Instill in ears
OU	Both eyes
p	After
p.c.	After meals
per	By, with
PO	By mouth
prn	As needed
q	Each
qh	Every hour
q2h	Every 2 hours
q6h	Every 6 hours
qid	4 times a day
qs	Quantity sufficient
Rx	Prescription
s	Without
sig	Label
ss	½
STAT	Immediately
tid	3 times a day

Drug Laws

Pure Food and Drug Act (1906)

- This was the first drug law passed in the United States.
- It ensures consumer quality (protects from imitations and false claims).
- It requires labeling to include ingredients and warnings.
- It sets U.S. standards for making each drug.
  - The United States Pharmacopeia and the National Formulary (USP-NF) comprise the official source of drug standards in the United States. This source describes approved medications and chemical formulas for approved drugs.

Federal Food, Drug, and Cosmetic Act of 1938

- This law gives the Food and Drug Administration (FDA) authority to oversee the safety of drugs (and food and cosmetics). The FDA is an agency of the Department of Health and Human Services.
- New products must be FDA approved.
- Prescription (Rx) and non-Rx drugs must be shown to be effective and safe.
- Drug utilization review is required.
- It includes regulations to prevent tampering.
- It requires accurate labels with the generic name included.
- It requires warning labels.

Controlled Substances Act (1970)

- This law was enacted to help reduce the abuse of legal and illegal drugs.
- A prescriber must register with the Drug Enforcement Agency (DEA), obtain a DEA registration number, and renew the registration annually.
- The law is enforced by the DEA through the Department of Justice.

Controlled Drugs

- Legal controlled drugs include those that require an Rx because of their potential for dependence, abuse, and addiction (e.g., depressants, stimulants, psychedelics, narcotics, anabolic steroids).
  - **Physical dependence:** A patient's reliance on a medication to relieve shaking, pain, or other symptoms
  - **Psychological dependence:** A patient's reliance on a medication to relieve anxiety, stress, tension, or other undesirable mental state
- The medical facility's on-site responsibilities are to:
  - Maintain a 2-year inventory of controlled drug transactions.
  - Securely store all Rx forms at a facility.
  - Keep a current drug reference book available at all times.
  - Keep controlled substances locked securely (double locked).

Drug Schedule

The Department of Justice places drugs into specific categories (schedules) according to their potential for abuse and dependence.

- **Schedule I**
  - Drugs with:
    - A high abuse and addiction potential
    - No medicinal use or no accepted safety for use (e.g., heroin, mescaline, or lysergic acid diethylamide [LSD])
- **Schedule II**
  - Drugs with:
    - A high abuse and addiction potential
    - A medicinal use (e.g., cocaine, morphine, methadone, codeine, Nembutal, Percodan, or Tylox)
  - A registered (DEA-licensed) provider must sign the Rx.
  - The Rx must be furnished to the pharmacy within 72 hours.

- If a schedule II drug is stored in a medical facility, it must be locked, routinely counted, and inventoried, and a dispensing record is kept for 2 years.
- **Schedule III**
  - These are drugs with a lower physical dependence but high psychological dependence potential (e.g., drugs with a limited amount of cocaine, narcotics, or amphetamine-like substances such as barbiturates, amphetamine compounds, paregoric, or Fiorinal).
  - The Rx is handwritten.
  - No DEA number is required.
  - Up to 5 refills in 6 months may be prescribed.
- **Schedule IV**
  - These are drugs with a lower abuse potential than schedule III drugs (e.g., mild tranquilizers and hypnotics such as diazepam, Librium, Valium, or Ambien).
  - The Rx may be written by an MA or RN, but it must be signed by an MD.
  - Up to 5 refills in 6 months may be prescribed, and it may be refilled by phone.
- **Schedule V**
  - These drugs require a written or oral Rx (e.g., drugs with a lower codeine level such as Lomotil, Robitussin A-C).
  - Orders and refills are the same as in schedule IV.

Drug References

United States Pharmacopeia and National Formulary (USP-NF)

- This is the official source of information for drugs approved by the FDA.
- It describes drug identification, strength, quality, and purity.
- It is updated every 5 years.

United States Pharmacopeia Dispensing Information (USP-DI)

- Electronic versions are updated each quarter.

- It contains 2 volumes:
  - Volume 1 is for prescribers. It contains industry-respected drug information (e.g., drug categories, indications, precautions, dosage forms).
  - Volume 2 is advice for the patient. It is written in lay person language and explains proper use of medication, description, precautions, side effects, and so forth.

Physicians' Drug Reference (PDR)

- This is the most comprehensive and widely used reference.
- This reference is organized into 6 sections:

  Section 1 (white): Manufacturers' index

  Section 2 (pink): Alphabetical arrangement of generic and brand-name index

  Section 3 (blue): Classification index

  Section 4 (gray): Manufacturers' photographic index displaying medications

  Section 5 (white): Product information

  Section 6 (white): Controlled-substance categories, poison control centers, drug information centers, sound-alike and look-alike drug names, and so forth

- Section 5 provides detailed information for each drug.
  - Actions
    - Descriptions of the cellular changes resulting from drug usage
    - Descriptions of the principal organ sites of actions
  - Cautions
    - Particular risks of using the drug, adverse reactions, and other side effects
    - Warnings and when to discontinue use
  - Contraindications
    - Conditions for which drug administration would be improper and/or undesirable
  - Indications
    - Conditions for which a drug is meant to be used

- Interactions
  - Other drugs or foods causing interactions that alter a drug's effect
  - Types of drug interactions:

Antagonism: This occurs when the presence of 1 drug decreases the intensity or shortens the duration of another drug's effect.

Potentiation: This occurs when 2 drugs are taken together and 1 of them exaggerates the action of the other. Example: An antihistamine taken with a painkilling narcotic intensifies the narcotic's effect; therefore, a reduced amount of narcotic is needed. This may be expressed as $a + n = N$.

Synergism: This is similar to potentiation. If 2 drugs are taken together that are similar in action (e.g., barbiturates and alcohol, which are both depressants), the combined effect is greater than the effect produced if each drug were taken separately. This may be expressed as $1 + 1 = 5$.

Common Drug Interactions

Several drugs are known to interact with specific substances and have potentially serious consequences.

Medication	Interactive Substances	Interaction Results
Hypoglycemic drugs—used to lower blood glucose level of diabetic patients	Alcohol or sulfonamide antibacterial drugs	Further lowering of blood sugar level; risk of severe hypoglycemia **(synergism)**
Depressants of central nervous system (CNS): sedatives, narcotic analgesics, antihistamines, alcohol	Any CNS depressants listed at left	Dangerous oversedation and respiratory failure **(synergism)**

Medication	Interactive Substances	Interaction Results
Anticoagulants	Aspirin, nonsteroidal anti-inflammatory drugs, alcohol, or antibiotics	Increased anticoagulant effect and risk of abnormal bleeding **(potentiation)**
Certain types of tetracycline antibiotics	Iron supplements, milk, or antacids	Reduced effectiveness of antibiotics if taken within 1 hour before or 2 hours after the antibiotics **(antagonism)**
Oral contraceptives	Barbiturates or some types of antibiotics	Reduced effectiveness of contraceptive and increased risk of pregnancy **(antagonism)**
Monoamine oxidase inhibitor antidepressants	Meperidine, decongestants, amphetamines, cheese, bananas, red wine, beer, yeast extract, or chocolate	Dangerous rise in blood pressure and risk of seizures or brain hemorrhage **(potentiation)**

Drug Names

Generic or Official	Trade or Brand	Chemical
Common or general name given when the drug is first produced Usually based on the chemical name Name not protected by trademark Drug less costly	Name that, on FDA approval, the manufacturer gives the drug Name protected by trademark	Scientific molecular structure of the drug (long and complicated)

Example: Tylenol is a trade name for acetaminophen, which is the generic name for the molecular compound N-Acetyl-p-aminophenol. Look and you will see acetaminophen and Tylenol within the chemical name.

FDA, Food and Drug Administration.

Drug Actions

Drug Effects

Local: Drug acts on the limited area to which it is administered (e.g., creams, numbing block).

Systemic: General effect. Drug is transported through the bloodstream and is carried to 1 or more tissues.

Drug Cycle Phases

Absorption	• Drug moves into the bloodstream from the site where it was administered
	• Rate at which drug passes from intestines into bloodstream and amount of drug passing into bloodstream (drug injection bypasses this stage) depend on the following:
	  • Drug form
	  • pH of medication
	  • Drug concentration
	  • Amount of food in stomach
	  • Depth of breathing for inhalants

Distribution	• Drug leaves bloodstream and passes into tissue spaces and cell bodies • Drug may pass across blood-brain barrier (this barrier regulates selection, degree, and rate of absorption into brain tissue) or placenta into fetus

Metabolism (biotransformation)	• Drug breakdown to another chemical within liver
	  • Usually results in inactivation of drug
	  • Sometimes converted to active form after liver absorption

Elimination	• Most common: Excretion in urine • Small amounts via saliva, sweat, stool, breast milk, breathing, and tears

Desired Effects of Drugs

Curative	To kill the causative factor of a condition or disease
Therapeutic	To relieve symptoms of disorder or disease
Destructive	To eliminate tumors and/or organisms
Palliative	To provide patient comfort; no cure; relieves pain or other symptoms
Prophylactic	To lessen severity of disease or prevent condition or disease
Replacement	To replace missing substances normally found in the body (e.g., hormones, vitamins)
Diagnostic	To test for allergies (antigen sera); radiographic studies (dye injection)

Factors Affecting Drug Action

Age
- Newborns are immature, and geriatric patients are deteriorating; both groups are sensitive to medications. Caution is used in dosage calculation.
- Geriatric patients: Metabolism, gastrointestinal function, drug sensitivity, hydration, safest route, psychosocial changes, and circulation are dosage considerations.
- Adult patients: Dosage calculation is based on age (20 to 60 years old) and weight (average 150 lb).
- Child patients: Dosage is usually calculated on the basis of mg of drug/kg of body weight. The body surface area is considered in calculation.

Body weight: The same dose of the same drug will have a lesser effect on a patient weighing more than on a patient weighing less.

Cumulation: Accumulation of the drug in the body resulting in toxicity. The drug has a much greater effect and toxic side effects. It usually results from a lack of elimination between administrations. Other factors are weight, age, sex, environment, psychological, genetics, and allergies.

Disease: Kidney and liver disease affects a drug's action. A drug's action may also begin the disease process affecting body organs.

Drug-drug interaction: One drug may potentiate or lessen the action of another drug.

Immune responses: A drug may cause a body to develop antibodies, and any future administration of the same drug would produce an allergic reaction.

Sex: Pregnant women, other women, and men are all affected differently by drugs. Intramuscular (IM) medications are absorbed more quickly by men than by women. Caution must be used with drug administration to pregnant women so as not to affect the fetus.

Tolerance: Reduced responsiveness to a drug. Tolerance may be inherited or acquired by use of the drug over a length of time.

Unintended Effects

Adverse reactions: These include ototoxicity, tinnitus, photosensitivity, and nephrotoxicity.

Toxic effects: These poisonous effects are the result of idiosyncrasies, a single overdose, or accumulation in blood levels over time.

Side effects: These are predictable reactions to a drug that can be expected to occur because of the way the drug works on different body tissues. Side effects are inevitable for most types of drugs. Some common side effects for several different drug groups are listed in the following table.

Drug Group	Common Side Effects
Angiotensin-converting enzyme (ACE) inhibitors	Dizziness, dry mouth, vomiting, cough, rash
Antibiotics	Diarrhea, thrush (a fungal infection, often in vagina), rash

Drug Group	Common Side Effects
Anticholinergic drugs	Blurred vision, dry mouth, urine retention
Antidepressants	Drowsiness, dry mouth, blurred vision, constipation
Antihistamines	Dizziness, drowsiness, clumsiness
Barbiturates	Dizziness, drowsiness, clumsiness
Benzodiazepines	Dizziness, drowsiness
Beta blockers	Wheezing, cold hands and feet, impotence
Cytotoxic anticancer drugs	Hair loss, diarrhea, vomiting, sores in the mouth
Narcotic analgesics	Constipation, nausea, vomiting, drowsiness
Nonsteroidal anti-inflammatory drugs (NSAIDs)	Indigestion, nausea, diarrhea, black bowel movements
Thiazide diuretics	Sensitivity to light, impotence
Vasodilators	Dizziness, fainting, ankle swelling

Drug Classifications

Trade Name	Generic Name	Used for or Actions
Analgesics		
Tylenol With Codeine	Acetaminophen and codeine	Pain reliever, antipyretic
Endocet	Oxycodone/APAP	Pain reliever, narcotic
Aleve	Naproxen	Nonopioid pain reliever, NSAID, antipyretic
Novocain (topical)	Procaine	Numbing local topical area

Continued

Trade Name	Generic Name	Used for or Actions
Xylocaine	Lidocaine 0.5% injection	Localized numbing
OxyContin	Oxycodone	Chronic moderate or severe pain relief of more than a few days
Percocet, Roxicet	Oxycodone/ acetaminophen	Pain reliever, narcotic
Ultram	Tramadol hydrochloride	Moderate pain relief, non-narcotic
Neurontin	Gabapentin	Nerve pain
Antiallergy Agents		
Allegra	Fexofenadine	Seasonal allergic rhinitis, chronic idiopathic urticaria, antihistamine
Atarax	Hydroxyzine hydrochloride	Antihistamine, antiemetic
Clarinex	Desloratadine	Seasonal allergies, H_1 histamine antagonist
Hydrocodone	Hydrocodone bitartrate	Antitussive for nonproductive dry cough, narcotic
Zyrtec	Cetirizine	Seasonal or perennial allergic rhinitis, chronic idiopathic urticaria, pruritus reduction, hives
Antibiotics		
Amoxicillin	Amoxicillin	Anti-infective, systemic chronic or acute infections
Amoxil	Amoxicillin	Anti-infective, acute or chronic systemic infections; also antiulcer, ENT infection

Trade Name	Generic Name	Used for or Actions
Augmentin	Amoxicillin-clavulanate	Soft tissue infection, moderate to severe bacterial infections, otitis media, sinusitis, UTI
Bactrim	Trimethoprim-sulfamethoxazole	UTI, URI, otitis media
Biaxin	Clarithromycin	Mild to moderate URI, chronic bronchitis, uncomplicated skin infections
Cefzil	Cefprozil	*Streptococcus* and *Staphylococcus* causing URI and skin infections
Cipro	Ciprofloxacin	UTI, URI, bone or joint infection, otitis media, skin infections
Flagyl	Metronidazole	Bacterial infections, stops parasites
Vibramycin, Doryx	Doxycycline	Bacterial infections, stops parasites, acne, venereal diseases, early Lyme disease, malaria preventive
Anticoagulants		
Aspirin	Aspirin or ASA (acetylsalicylic acid)	Blood thinner, analgesic, antipyretic
Coumadin	Warfarin	Clotting disorders, myocardial infarction, chronic atrial fibrillation, blood thinner
Antiarrhythmic Agents		
Dilantin	Phenytoin	Anticonvulsant
Lanoxin	Digoxin	Slows and strengthens heartbeat, hypertension

Continued

Trade Name	Generic Name	Used for or Actions
Antidepressants		
Paxil	Paroxetine hydrochloride	Depression, anxiety, panic disorder
Ativan	Lorazepam	Anxiety
Celexa	Citalopram	Depression, anxiety
Lexapro	Escitalopram	Depression, anxiety
Wellbutrin XL	Bupropion hydrochloride	Depression
Zoloft	Sertraline hydrochloride	Depression, obsessive-compulsive disorder
Xanax	Alprazolam	Anxiety, panic disorders
Antidiabetic Agents		
Avandia	Rosiglitazone maleate	NIDDM (type 2 diabetes)
Glucophage	Metformin	NIDDM (type 2 diabetes)
Glucotrol XL	Glipizide	NIDDM (type 2 diabetes)
Antifungal Agents		
Diflucan	Fluconazole	Oropharyngeal, vaginal, and systemic candidiasis
Mycostatin	Nystatin	*Candida* skin and mucous membrane infections
Antihyperlipidemic Agents		
Lipitor	Atorvastatin calcium	Reduction of cholesterol levels
Pravachol	Pravastatin sodium	Reduction of cholesterol levels

Trade Name	Generic Name	Used for or Actions
Zocor	Simvastatin	Reduction of triglycerides (LDL)
Crestor	Rosuvastatin	Reduction of cholesterol levels
Vytorin	Ezetimibe and simvastatin	Reduction of cholesterol levels
Antihypertensive Agents		
Accupril	Quinapril hydrochloride	Hypertension, CHF, ACE inhibitor
Cozaar	Losartan potassium	Hypertension
Lasix	Furosemide	Hypertension, CHF, diuretic for edema
Lotensin	Benazepril hydrochloride	Hypertensive
Metoprolol	Hydrochlorothiazide (HCTZ)	Hypertension, diuretic for edema
Norvasc	Amlodipine besylate	Hypertension, angina, calcium channel blocker
Prinivil	Lisinopril	Hypertension, angina, ACE inhibitor
Toprol XL	Metoprolol succinate	Hypertension, angina pectoris
Zestril	Lisinopril	Hypertensive, ACE inhibitor, CHF
Anti-inflammatory Agents		
Aleve	Naproxen	Arthritis, dysmenorrhea
Celebrex	Celecoxib	Pain associated with arthritis

Continued

Trade Name	Generic Name	Used for or Actions
Antiulcer Agents		
Prevacid	Lansoprazole	Short-term treatment for active duodenal ulcer, gastric ulcer, erosive esophagitis
Prilosec	Omeprazole	Gastric and duodenal ulcers, GERD
Bronchodilators		
Aminophylline	Theophylline ethylenediamine	Bronchospasm prevention and symptom relief
Epi-EZ Pen, Primatene Mist Suspension	Epinephrine	Temporary relief of bronchospasm from asthma, anaphylactic reactions
Proventil HFA	Albuterol	Prevention of bronchospasm associated with asthma, bronchitis
Corticosteroids		
Flonase	Fluticasone	Seasonal or perennial allergic and nonallergic rhinitis
Nasonex	Mometasone furoate	Steroid-dependent asthma, seasonal or perennial allergic rhinitis
Deltasone	Prednisone	Arthritis, blood disorders, breathing problems, severe allergies
Hormones		
Climara	Estradiol	Contraceptive, HRT
Humulin N insulin	Isophane insulin, human rDNA	Hyperglycemia, IDDM (type 1 diabetes)

Trade Name	Generic Name	Used for or Actions
Humalog KwikPen U-100 Insulin Pen	Insulin lispro	Hyperglycemia, IDDM (type 1 diabetes)
Novolin N Flexpen U-100	Insulin NPH isophane human	Hyperglycemia, IDDM (type 1 diabetes)
Premarin	Estrogen	Imbalance: breast and prostate, osteoporosis, menopausal symptoms
Synthroid	Levothyroxine	Hypothyroidism, cretinism, myxedema
Hypnotics/Sedatives		
Ambien	Zolpidem tartrate	Insomnia
Lunesta	Eszopiclone	Insomnia
Oleptro ER	Trazodone	Major depression, insomnia associated with depression
Supplements and Replacements		
Fosamax	Alendronate	Treatment and prevention of osteoporosis in postmenopausal women
Klor-Con	Potassium chloride	Hypokalemia, electrolyte supplement
Levoxyl	Levothyroxine	Treatment of low thyroid function (hypothyroidism)

ACE, angiotensin-converting enzyme; APAP, acetaminophen; CHF, congestive heart failure; ENT, ear, nose, and throat; GERD, gastroesophageal reflux disease; HRT, hormone replacement therapy; IDDM, insulin-dependent diabetes mellitus; LDL, low-density lipoprotein; NIDDM, non–insulin dependent diabetes mellitus; NSAID, nonsteroidal anti-inflammatory drug; URI, upper respiratory infection; UTI, urinary tract infection.

The "7 Rights" for Drug Administration

Patients receiving medications should always feel safe. Checking and observing each of the following items ensure error elimination in medication preparation and administration.

Right dose	Check the amount of drug and correct strength
Right drug	Check label 3 times 1. On removal from storage 2. While preparing 3. On return to storage
Right technique	Administer the drug using the correct method and at the correct site
Right route	Administer the drug using the correct route: oral, topical, parenteral, optic, or ophthalmic
Right time	Administer the drug at the correct time; some patients should be told when the next dose is due
Right patient	Know the patient to whom the drug is to be administered (verify patient's full name and date of birth)
Right documentation (the medical record is a legal document)	4. Patient's name 5. Date and time of administration 6. Drug name and dosage given 7. Route used, site if injected, and any complications 8. Any adverse reactions 9. Reasons for not administering 10. Signed by the medical assistant

Prescription Components (Legend)

- Written by an MD and filled by a pharmacist
- Indicates medication needed and includes all directions for the pharmacist and patient
- Contains the following:
  - Name of drug

- Dosage (the amount of medicine prescribed for administration)
- When drug is to be given
- How it is given
- How many times it is given
- Date of the order
- Signature of MD who wrote it

Inscription: Name of drug, dosage, form, and strength

Superscription: Patient's name and address, date, and the symbol Rx (means "take")

Subscription: Number of doses dispensed and quantities

Sig. (signature): Directions for taking the drug, usually preceded by the term Sig. (means "mark")

Drug Delivery Systems

Oral

The route is convenient, safe, and relatively inexpensive. Most drugs are taken 1 to 2 hours after meals.

Solid Forms

Caplet: Shaped like a capsule but with the consistency of a tablet

Capsule: A 2-part container: shell dissolves in the gastrointestinal tract; drug-embedded powder or beads contained inside

Tablet: Compressed powder; various shapes, colors; may be **enteric**-coated, scored, or layered

Liquid Forms

Elixir: Solution containing sugar, alcohol, and water

Emulsion: Fine droplets of fat globules in water (homogenized milk)

Solution: Liquid homogeneous preparation containing 1 or more substances; combination made up of a **solute** (dissolved substance) and a **solvent** (liquid in which solute is dissolved)

Spirit: Solution containing alcohol

Suspension: Drug particles suspended within a liquid, not dissolved

Syrup: Liquids containing sugar (e.g., ipecac)

Tincture: Solution of drug(s) dissolved in alcohol with or without water

Topical

Liniment: Drug mixed with oil, soap, water, or alcohol. It is used externally on skin to produce warmth in the area where drug is needed.

Lotion: Suspension or emulsion preparation. It is used externally on skin in the area where drug is needed.

Ointment: Salve with fatty base (petroleum jelly, lanolin, lard). It is applied externally to skin in the area where drug is needed.

Transdermal

Medication is typically contained in an adhesive patch or disk attached to the skin. The patch allows a slow controlled delivery *through* the skin to deeper tissue or the circulation system. Examples of patch drugs include estrogen, nitroglycerin, and nicotine.

Mucous Membrane

Selected membranes absorb medication for a systemic effect.

Suppository

This form is designed to melt after insertion; it is used **rectally, vaginally,** or in **urethra.** (The patient should be in **Sims' position** for rectal suppository insertion.)

Ophthalmic

- **Eye ointment:** The tip allows dispensing of a small stream into the bottom eyelid.

- **Eyedrops:** They are placed in the center of the lower conjunctival sac.

Buccal

Medication is in tablet or gum form; absorption is through the gums and cheeks. Do not chew.

Sublingual

The preparation is placed under the tongue; it is dissolved and then absorbed.

Inhalation

Nasal or mouth membrane delivery occurs through atomizers or inhalers. The drug is suspended as tiny droplets in an aerosol form.

Otic (ear)

- Although the ear is not a mucous membrane, the drop form is common for otic medication instillation.
- **Drop instillation:** For adults, pull the pinna up and back. For children younger than 3 years old, pull the lobe down and back.

Parenteral (Injection)

- Parenteral administration is used when a drug cannot be given orally, through a mucous membrane, or topically.
- Administering drugs by injection is the surest and fastest method of drug delivery to the body.
- The risk of overdosing is higher.
- Effectiveness is determined by the site's blood supply.

Needle Gauges

- Gauges are determined by the size of the needle lumen (diameter of opening).
- The higher the gauge number, the smaller the lumen is.

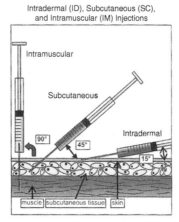

Intradermal (ID), Subcutaneous (SC),
and Intramuscular (IM) Injections

ID, SC, and IM angles of injection. *Courtesy of Myers, E, and Hopkins, T: MedSurg Notes, F.A. Davis, 2004.*

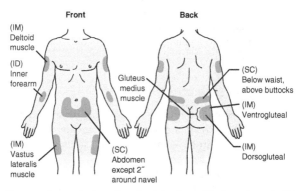

Commonly used sites for the injection: ID, intradermal; IM, intramuscular; SC, subcutaneous.

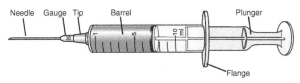

The parts of a syringe.

Types of Injections

- **Intravenous (IV):** instantaneous effect
- **Intradermal (ID)**
  - Bevel up, do not aspirate. This is used for the purified protein derivative (PPD) tuberculin test.
- **Subcutaneous (SC)**
  1. Grasp skin to form a 1-inch fold.
  2. Aspirate.
  3. Inject slowly.
- For insulin injection:
  1. Roll the vial between palms to mix evenly.
  2. Do not shake.
  3. Do not massage after injection (also true in administering Imferon, heparin).
- **Intramuscular (IM):** Faster effect than SC
  1. Stretch skin taut.
  2. Aspirate.
  3. Inject slowly.
  4. Cover the site.
  5. Massage.
- **"Z-track"** injection:
  1. Pull skin 1.5 inch away from the injection site.
  2. Insert at a 90° angle in a dartlike fashion.
  3. Aspirate.
  4. Inject slowly.
  5. Wait 10 seconds before withdrawing; remove the needle at the same angle, and release skin.
  6. Do not massage.

Text continued on page 304

Immunizations

Recommended Adult Immunization Schedule by Age Group United States, 2019

Vaccine	19–21 years	22–26 years	27–49 years	50–64 years	≥65 years
Influenza inactivated (IIV) or Influenza recombinant (RIV)	1 dose annually				
Influenza live attenuated (LAIV)			1 dose annually		
Tetanus, diphtheria, pertussis (Tdap or Td)	1 dose Tdap, then Td booster every 10 yrs				
Measles, mumps, rubella (MMR)	1 or 2 doses depending on indication (if born in 1957 or later)				
Varicella (VAR)	2 doses (if born in 1980 or later)				
Zoster recombinant (RZV) (preferred)				2 doses	
Zoster live (ZVL)					1 dose

Recommended vaccination for adults who meet age requirement, lack documentation of vaccination, or lack evidence of past infection

Recommended vaccination for adults with an additional risk factor or another indication

No recommendation

Recommended Adult Immunization Schedule by Age Group United States, 2019

Vaccine	19–21 years	22–26 years	27–49 years	50–64 years	≥65 years
Human papillomavirus (HPV) Female	2 or 3 doses depending on age at initial vaccination				
Human papillomavirus (HPV) Male	2 or 3 doses depending on age at initial vaccination				
Pneumococcal conjugate (PCV13)				1 dose	
Pneumococcal polysaccharide (PPSV23)	1 or 2 doses depending on indication				1 dose
Hepatitis A (HepA)	2 or 3 doses depending on vaccine				
Hepatitis B (HepB)	2 or 3 doses depending on vaccine				
Meningococcal A, C, W, Y (MenACWY)	1 or 2 doses depending on indication, then booster every 5 yrs if risk remains				
Meningococcal B (MenB)	2 or 3 doses depending on vaccine and indication				
Haemophilus influenzae type b (Hib)	1 or 3 doses depending on indication				

Recommended vaccination for adults who meet age requirement, lack documentation of vaccination, or lack evidence of past infection

Recommended vaccination for adults with an additional risk factor or another indication

No recommendation

Continued

Recommended Adult Immunization Schedule by Medical Condition and Other Indications United States, 2019

Vaccine	Pregnancy	Immuno-com-promised (excluding HIV infection)	HIV infection CD4 count <200	HIV infection CD4 count ≥200	Asplenia, comple-ment deficien-cies	End-stage renal disease, on hemo-dialysis	Heart or lung disease, alcoholism	Chronic liver disease	Diabetes	Health care personnel[2]	Men who have sex with men
IIV or RIV	1 dose annually										
LAIV	1 dose annually										
Tdap or Td	1 dose Tdap each pregnancy	1 dose Tdap, then Td booster every 10 yrs									
MMR	CONTRAINDICATED	CONTRAINDICATED	CONTRAINDICATED		1 or 2 doses depending on indication						
VAR	CONTRAINDICATED	CONTRAINDICATED	CONTRAINDICATED		2 doses						
RZV (preferred)	DELAY				2 doses at age ≥50 yrs						
ZVL	CONTRAINDICATED	CONTRAINDICATED			1 dose at age ≥60 yrs						

Legend:
- Recommended vaccination for adults who meet age requirement, lack documentation of vaccination, or lack evidence of past infection
- Recommended vaccination for adults with an additional risk factor or another indication
- Precaution—vaccine might be indicated if benefit of protection outweighs risk of adverse reaction
- Delay vaccination until after pregnancy if vaccine is indicated
- Contraindicated—vaccine should not be administered because of risk for serious adverse reaction
- No recommendation

PRECAUTION

1. Precaution for LAIV does not apply to alcoholism. 2. See notes for influenza; hepatitis B; measles, mumps, and rubella; and varicella vaccinations.
3. Hematopoietic stem cell transplant.

Recommended Adult Immunization Schedule by Medical Condition and Other Indications United States, 2019

Vaccine	Pregnancy	Immuno-compromised (excluding HIV infection)	HIV infection CD4 count <200	HIV infection CD4 count ≥200	Asplenia complement deficiencies	End-stage renal disease, on hemo-dialysis	Heart or lung disease, alcoholism	Chronic liver disease	Diabetes	Health care personnel [2]	Men who have sex with men
HPV Female	DELAY	3 doses through age 26 yrs									2 or 3 doses through age 26 yrs
HPV Male		3 doses through age 26 yrs			2 or 3 doses through age 21 yrs						2 or 3 doses through age 26 yrs
PCV13						1 dose					
PPSV23				1, 2, or 3 doses depending on age and indication							
HepA				2 or 3 doses depending on vaccine							
HepB				2 or 3 doses depending on vaccine							
MenACWY		1 or 2 doses depending on indication, then booster every 5 yrs if risk remains									
MenB	PRECAUTION			2 or 3 doses depending on vaccine and indication							
Hib		3 doses HSCT[3] recipients only			1 dose						

Recommended vaccination for adults who meet age requirement, lack documentation of vaccination, or lack evidence of past infection

Recommended vaccination for adults with an additional risk factor or another indication

Precaution—vaccine might be indicated if benefit of protection outweighs risk of adverse reaction

Delay vaccination until after pregnancy if vaccine is indicated

Contraindicated—vaccine should not be administered because of risk for serious adverse reaction

No recommendation

1. Precaution for LAIV does not apply to alcoholism. 2. See notes for influenza; hepatitis B; measles, mumps, and rubella; and varicella vaccinations.
3. Hematopoietic stem cell transplant.

Metric and Household Measurements

Common Metric Prefixes

Unit(s)	Prefix	Decimal Form
1,000	Kilo	1,000
100	Hecto	100
10	Deka	10
1/10 of a unit	Deci	0.1
1/100 of a unit	Centi	0.01
1/1,000 of a unit	Milli	0.001
1/1,000,000 of a unit	Micro	0.000001

Most Often Used Abbreviations

Metric		Household	
Milliliter	mL	Ounce	oz
Liter	L	Pound	lb
Cubic centimeter	cc	Teaspoon	tsp
Grain	gr	Tablespoon	tbsp
Microgram	mcg	Pint	pt
Milligram	mg	Quart	qt
Gram	g (gm also used)	Gallon	gal
Kilogram	kg	Inch	in"
Millimeter	mm		
Centimeter	cm		
Meter	m		

Metric System

Length: Measured in meters (m)
100 centimeters (cm) = 1 meter (m)

Volume (fluids): Measured in liters (L)
1,000 milliliters (mL) = 1 liter (L)
Weight (solids): Measured in grams (g)
1,000 micrograms (mcg) = 1 milligram (mg)
1,000 milligrams (mg) = 1 gram (g)
1,000 grams (g) = 1 kilogram (kg)

To Convert Metric Weight

mg to g: Divide by 1,000, or move the decimal point 3 places
   to the left.
g to mg: Multiply by 1,000, or move the decimal point
   3 places to the right.
g to kg: Divide by 1,000, or move the decimal point 3 places
   to the left.
kg to g: Multiply by 1,000, or move the decimal point 3 places
   to the right.

To Convert Metric Volume

L to mL: Multiply by 1,000, or move the decimal point 3
   places to the right.
mL to L: Divide by 1,000, or move the decimal point 3 places
   to the left.

Approximate Equivalents to Household Measures

- **Volume**
  1 teaspoon (tsp) = 5 mL
  1 tablespoon (tbsp) = 15 mL
  1 ounce (oz) = 30 mL
  1 cup (8 oz) = 240 mL
  1 pint = 500 mL
  1 quart = 1,000 mL, 1,000 cc (also cm^3)
- **Weight**
  1 oz = 30 g
  16 oz = 1 pound (lb)
  2.2 lb = 1 kg
- **Length**
  2.5 cm = 1 inch (in$''$)

Temperature Conversion

- Formula to convert Fahrenheit (F) to Celsius (C):

$$C = (F - 32) \times 5/9$$

  1. Subtract 32 from the Fahrenheit temperature.
  2. Multiply the result by 5.
  3. Divide the result by 9.
- Formula to convert Celsius (C) to Fahrenheit (F):

$$F = 9 \times C \div 5 + 32$$

  1. Multiply C by 9.
  2. Divide the result by 5.
  3. Add 32 to the result.

Dosing Calculation Formula

- Use the ratio proportion method to solve for X (simple algebra).
- A ratio is a way to show the relationship between the numerator and the denominator of a fraction.
- A proportion is the comparison of 2 ratios.

Sample problem to solve: 3,600 mg = g

1. Set up your equation to have X represent your unknown.
2. To the left of the equal sign (=) set up the equivalent measure you know.

$$1,000 \text{ mg} : 1 \text{ g}$$

(This is the known ratio relationship.)

3. Follow the same sequence on the right side of the equal sign (=) that you used on the left, and insert the X for the unknown you are looking for:

$$1,000 \text{ mg} : 1 \text{ g} = 3,600 \text{ mg} : X \text{ g}$$

(This is proportion showing the relationship between ratios.)

4. The proportion method uses the terms *means* and *extremes*.

   In this case, the means are 1 g and 3,600 mg.

   The extremes are 1,000 mg and X g.

You will always know either both your means or both your extremes.

5. Multiply together the known means or extremes. In this case, both means are known.

$$1 \times 3,600$$

6. Take the answer (which is 3,600) and divide by the 1 known extreme.

$$1,000$$

7. Your answer should be: X = **3.6 g**

Another sample problem to solve: 4 mg : 50 lb = X mg : 150 lb

1. Both extremes are known.

$$4 \text{ and } 150$$

2. Multiply them:

$$600$$

3. Divide by the known mean:

$$50$$

4. Your answer should be: X = **12 mg**

YOUR NOTES

_____

_____

_____

_____

_____

_____

_____

Additional Vocabulary

Ampule: Small, prefilled glass container holding a sterile solution or powder; container has a scored neck and is designed for 1 use only

Aspirate: A step in the injection process; to pull back on the hypodermic plunger to ensure that the needle is not in blood vessel; no blood should be present in the needle barrel; failing to aspirate may deliver an IM or SC injection as an IV injection

Average dose: Most effective with minimum toxic effect

Cartridge-needle unit: Holds premeasured medication; disposed of after use

Cumulative dose: The total amount of medication present in the body after repeated dosing

Dispense: Prepare and give a medication to patient

Divided dose: A smaller measured portion given at shorter intervals

Enteric-coated: Drug form designed to bypass stomach to then dissolve in intestine

Initial dose: The first dose

Maintenance dose: Amount needed for the drug to remain at therapeutic level in bloodstream

Maximum dose: Largest amount given that is safe

Medication unit: Expresses potency of drugs too varied in their potency (insulin)

Minimum dose: The smallest amount that will still be effective

Pharmacodynamics: The analysis of a drug's effect on living organisms

Pharmacokinetics: Study of drug actions and metabolism within the body

Prescribe: Recommend or order therapeutic treatment or use of a drug

Toxic dose: Amount causing signs and symptoms of drug poisoning

Vial: Prefilled small glass container holding sterile solution or powder; rubber stopped for needle entry

Viscosity: Liquid thickness and stickiness

Wheal: Slight elevation of skin; the result of ID injection

YOUR NOTES

_____

_____

_____

_____

_____

_____

Sample Certification Test Questions

Now that you have studied this chapter, here are some sample certification test questions for you.

1. Which of the following is not an antidiabetic agent?

   A. Glucotrol XL
   B. Avandia
   C. Glucophage
   D. Premarin
   E. All are diabetic agents

2. The MD orders dimenhydrinate liquid 50 mg PO. The stock container is labeled 12.5 mg/1 mL. How much medication should be given to the patient?

   A. 2 mL
   B. 3 mL
   C. 3.5 mL
   D. 4 mL
   E. 4.5 mL

3. Sensitivity to light and impotence may become side effects of

   A. Antibiotic agents
   B. Thiazide agents
   C. Antispasmodic agents
   D. Antidepressant agents
   E. Antiemetic agents

See the Appendix for the answers.

DAVIS
edge.

Remember to use Edge after you finish this chapter to test your knowledge. Directions for how to access Edge, as well as your access code, are located on the inside front cover of this text.

Chapter 10

Laboratory Diagnostics

Laboratory testing is an important part of patient care. In an outpatient setting, medical assistants can perform Clinical Laboratory Improvement Amendments (CLIA)–waived tests. These tests include laboratory analysis of heart function, respiration, urine, blood, and other bodily fluids, which provide needed information about the patient's health. Testing can identify diagnoses and can monitor the patient's response to dosing of various medications.

This chapter helps you review the laboratory content you may encounter on the examination. This content includes common abbreviations, laboratory safety, quality control, the microscope, microbiology, specimen collection and handling, urinalysis, hematology, venipuncture, serology, the cardiac cycle and electrocardiograms (ECGs), pulmonary function testing, and radiology information.

Remember to use Edge after you finish this chapter to test your knowledge. Directions for how to access Edge, as well as your access code, are located on the inside front cover of this text.

Common Abbreviations

Abbreviation	Meaning
bx, bi	Biopsy
CBC	Complete blood count
C&S	Culture and sensitivity
DNA	Deoxyribonucleic acid
EEG	Electroencephalogram

Continued

Abbreviation	Meaning
FBS	Fasting blood sugar
H&H, H/H	Hemoglobin and hematocrit
HCG	Human chorionic gonadotropin
POCT	Point-of-care testing
Pap	Papanicolaou test (Pap)
pH	Potential hydrogen
QRS	Ventricular depolarization
STAT	Immediately
STD	Sexually transmitted disease
TC	Throat culture
UA	Urinalysis
UC	Urine culture
U	Unit
mU	Milliunit

Laboratory Safety

Standard (Universal) Precautions

- Treat all blood and body fluids as infectious.
- Use personal protective equipment (PPE):
  - Sterile or nonsterile gloves, laboratory coat, shoe covers, and gown
  - Protective eyewear, mask, and face shield
- Protect patients from you; protect yourself from patients.
- Use special care to avoid injury from sharp instruments and equipment.
  - Never use needles or other sharps unnecessarily.
  - Dispose of sharps in puncture- and leak-proof containers.

- Report all accidental contaminated sharp injuries to supervisors.

Be sure to: Perform needed medical or surgical hand washing before clinical procedures and after patient contact.

Environment Safety

- Employee training in workplace hazards is supplied.
  - Provided at the time an employee begins work in which exposure may occur
  - Comprehensive review provided annually, or more often if needed
- An employer accidental-exposure plan must be in place.
  - Outlines protective measures used to eliminate or minimize exposure risk
  - Identifies employees with occupational exposure
  - Documents exposure, postexposure evaluation, and follow-up procedures for accidental exposure to potentially infectious materials
- Each hazardous substance must be identified with a hazardous label displaying the name of contained material and list effects of the chemical.
- Material Safety Data Sheets (MSDSs) are used for hazardous agents.
  - Available from the product manufacturer
  - Contain information about hazardous chemicals or other substances
- All puncture-proof sharps containers, biohazard bags, and eyewash stations must be correctly labeled.

Quality Control

The medical facility's procedure manual describes proper test processes, result reporting, and documentation. For example:

- Place specimen collected for pathological testing in formalin preservative; for microbiological culturing, treat as sterilely as possible, and do not expose to formalin.

- Give patients verbal and written procedure performance instructions, and confirm patients' understanding of procedure steps.
- Clinical employees receive refresher laboratory procedure training each year.

Quality Maintenance

- Check expiration dates of collection containers, tubes, swabs, reagents, and so forth before use.
- Calibrate laboratory instruments to ensure correct operation.
- Each calibration must be recorded in a quality-control log.
- Perform calibration routines on a set of standards alone.
  - A **standard** is a specimen like one you would normally process, except that the value for the standard is already known.
- Verify calibrations at least every 6 months.
- Perform and document control testing each day on appropriate tests.
- Control samples are used 1st every time a patient's sample is processed.
- Generally, positive and negative control samples are used with a test that yields a **qualitative test response** (substance tested for is either present or absent).
- Other control samples show when results fall within a normal range. These samples are used for tests that give **quantitative test results** (the concentration of a test substance in a specimen).
- When testing, adhere to procedures designed to identify problems with equipment calibration, errors in testing procedures, and defective testing supplies.
- Perform and document equipment maintenance: cleaning, adjusting, and part replacement.

The Microscope

This essential component of the laboratory illuminates and magnifies specimens so that they may be viewed and analyzed. It is a complex and delicate piece of equipment. It should not be moved around in the laboratory unless absolutely necessary. If it must be moved, grasp the arm and support the weight of the microscope at the base.

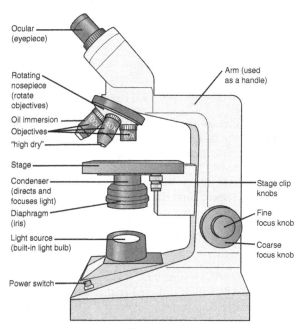

Microscope.

Microscope Components

- **Light source:** Usually a built-in light bulb located directly under the center of the stage
- **Ocular lens** (eyepiece)/**biocular lens** (eyepieces)
  - It is located at the top of the microscope.
  - It magnifies the field of view 10 times (10× lens).
- **Objectives:** Contain the magnifying lens
  - They are located at the center of the microscope just above the stage and mounted on a swivel base.

- Two objectives are dry (air between objective and pre-pared slide).
  - Dry lens magnifications are 10× (low power) and 40× (high power).
- One objective is oil-immersed (oil drop touches lens and prepared slide).
  - Oil-immersed object magnification is 100×.
- **Stage**
  - A prepared slide is placed here and held in place with metal clips.
  - An opening in stage allows light passage to a prepared slide.
- **Condenser**
  - On a substage (just below the stage), it directs and focuses the light through the slide.
  - The condenser can be raised and lowered.
- **Iris** (diaphragm)
  - It is located within the condenser.
  - It can be opened and closed to regulate the intensity of the light passing through the condenser.

Uses of the Microscope Objectives' Magnification

- Low power (10×) is used for:
  - Urine sediment for casts and epithelial cells
  - Scanning blood smears
- High power (40×) is used for:
  - Wet preparation: Urine sediment for red blood cells (RBCs), white blood cells (WBCs), bacteria, yeast, and parasites
- Oil immersion (100×) is used for:
  - Microorganisms
  - Blood films (blood cell morphology, count, WBC differential)

Microbiology

Microbiology is the study of minute unicellular, multicel-lular, and acellular organisms. The study includes the areas of bacteriology, virology, mycology, and parasitology. Most microorganisms residing on or in the body are called normal flora. Only a small number of microorganisms are pathogenic in the body and fall into the category of infectious disease.

Microorganisms: The major groups of microorganisms are bacteria, fungi, parasites, and archaea. Microorganisms are normally found almost everywhere: in our food and water, in the air, in soil, in the skin, and within the body.

Morphology: This is the study of form and structure of an organism and the special features specific to it.

Normal flora: The microorganisms found on skin and within the body that do not normally cause disease. Some are beneficial to the body, such as those that destroy potentially harmful microorganisms within the intestinal tract.

Pathogens: Microorganisms that cause disease. These infectious agents are capable of being transmitted from 1 living being to another in which they grow and multiply and causing infection without signs of disease.

Virulence: The capacity of a microorganism to cause illness.

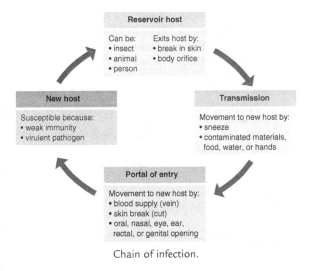

Chain of infection.

Bacteria

Bacteria are single-celled **(prokaryote)** organisms and are considered to be vegetable matter. Antibiotics effectively fight and control bacterial infections.

Classification

There are 4 ways that bacteria are identified:
- The conditions in which they thrive
  - **Aerobes** require oxygen (O_2) to survive.
  - **Anaerobes** do not require O_2; some types will die when exposed to O_2.
- **Morphology:** The form and shape of the organism
  - **Cocci** (round); singular, **coccus**
    - Cause such diseases as pneumonia, streptococcal throat, and gonorrhea
  - **Bacilli** (rod-shaped); singular, **bacillus**
    - Cause such diseases as tuberculosis (TB), tetanus, urinary tract infection (UTI), and whooping cough
  - **Spirilla** (spiral); singular, **spirillum**
    - Cause such diseases as syphilis and Lyme disease
  - **Staphylo;** grapelike clusters
    - Methicillin-resistant *Staphylococcus aureus* (MRSA) is a strain of staph bacteria that is resistant to prescribed antibiotics. MRSA most often occurs in people who have been in hospitals or health-care settings. If a disease, such as this, originated or is acquired in a hospital, it is referred to as a **nosocomial infection.**
  - Some bacteria may make **spores** (hard-shelled formations).
  - Spores are resistant to heat and disinfectants, thus making them difficult to kill.
  - Some bacteria may have **flagella** (projections enabling movement).
  - **Bacteria arrangements (and their associated prefixes)** include the following:
    - Chains = strepto-
    - Pirs = diplo-
    - Clusters = staphylo-

- The patterns of reproduction: A colony's appearance and patterns as it grows on a culture medium
  - Odor and color are also factors in identification.
- Staining
  - Stained slides are used to identify bacteria, most often with the Gram stain.
  - Staining divides bacteria into 3 groups:
    - **Gram-positive bacteria (purple):** Agents of botulism, diphtheria, pneumonia, rheumatic fever, staphylococcal infection, tetanus, and streptococcal throat
    - **Gram-negative bacteria (pink):** Agents of gonorrhea, meningitis, UTI, cholera, pertussis, plague, typhoid fever, and dysentery
    - Acid-fast staining: May be used if Gram staining does not stain the specimen sufficiently. This usually identifies bacteria with a waxy cell wall, such as the agent of tuberculosis.

Fungi

Fungi (singular form, fungus) are single-celled (eukaryote) organisms and are larger than bacteria. Fungal infections may produce disease in the heart, lungs, skin, hair, nails, and other organs. They are resistant to antibiotics.

- Yeasts are single-celled fungi.
- Molds are multicellular fungi that produce spores.
  - An important species of mold is *Penicillium*. The 1st antibiotic drug, penicillin, was developed from this mold.
- **Tinea:** A fungal skin infection. Types of tinea include the following:
  - Athlete's foot (tinea pedis)
  - Ringworm
  - Thrush (oral yeast)

Parasites

Parasites (protists) live on or in another organism (host). These are all eukaryotes that are not fungi, plants, or animals. Parasites include the causative agents of malaria, gastroenteritis,

African sleeping sickness, and amebic encephalitis. They are mostly single celled, have a nucleus, and prefer aquatic or moist environments. They use the other organism for their nourishment, growth, and reproduction. The host is harmed as the parasite thrives.

- Infection by a parasite is referred to as infestation.
  - Most parasites are identified in microscopic examination of urine, feces, tissue fluids, and biopsy specimens.
- Various parasites are as follows:
  - Worms (helminths): These include roundworms, whipworms, tapeworms, and pinworms.
  - Insects: These spread viral, bacterial, and protozoa diseases; such insects include mosquitoes, ticks, lice, and mites.
  - Single-celled protozoa: Protozoa cause such conditions as malaria and dysentery.

Archaea

These single-celled microorganisms are similar in size and shape to bacteria and have a wide variety of cell shapes. They can live in hostile environments and some interact with other organisms, but none are known to cause disease. They lack cell nuclei. They are prokaryotes.

Virology

Virology is the study of viruses. Virology is considered a subfield of microbiology because viruses are generally nonliving; therefore, they are not microorganisms. They are not made of cells, they do not grow, or make their own energy, and they cannot remain in a stable state. A virus is an infective agent consisting of proteins and genetic material (either DNA or RNA, but never both). Once a virus is within a living host cell, it is capable of copying itself and usually has a detrimental effect.

A virus relies on host cells to grow, reproduce, and then invade more host cells.

Most viral diseases can be treated only for the symptoms they produce in their hosts. Antibiotics are ineffective as treatment. The host must endure the disease until it has run its course (i.e., herpes, HIV infection, hepatitis, rubella, mumps, Ebola, rabies, influenza, common colds (coronaviruses), and shingles.

A **novel coronavirus** is a new coronavirus that has not been previously identified. Sometimes coronaviruses that infect animals can evolve to make people sick and become a new human coronavirus. Three examples are novel coronavirus 2019 (2019-nCoV), severe acute respiratory syndrome coronavirus (SARS-CoV), and Middle East respiratory syndrome coronavirus (MERS-CoV). Severe SARS-CoV is known as SARS-CoV-2, the cause of coronavirus disease 2019 (COVID-19).

- **Blood-borne viral infections**
  - These diseases live in the host's blood.
  - They are transmitted from host to host through contact with the infected body fluids, blood and blood products, or mucous membranes.
  - Other substances may also transmit the viral infection if they have traces of blood in them, such as vomitus, urine, sputum, feces, perspiration, tears, saliva, and nasal secretions.

Hepatitis Viruses

Hepatitis A virus (HAV)	Acute infective Transmitted by fecal or oral contamination
Hepatitis B virus (HBV)	Most common Infection transmitted through contaminated serum, plasma, needles, and entry through all entry portals
Hepatitis C virus (HCV)	Transmitted by blood transfusion or needle sharing

Continued

Hepatitis D virus (HDV)	Also known as delta hepatitis Occurs in patients with hepatitis B Transmitted by mucosal contact, needle sharing, and sexual contact
Hepatitis E virus (HEV)	Acute Occurs mostly outside the United States Transmitted by fecally contaminated water or food

Human Immunodeficiency Virus (HIV)

- Transmitted acutely:
  - Blood-to-blood and sexual contact are modes of transmission.
  - It may be present in all body fluids.
  - Of those infected, 70% will progress to **acquired immunodeficiency syndrome (AIDS).**

Stages of HIV Infection	
Stage 1	Acute HIV infection; patient becomes an HIV carrier
Stage 2	Asymptomatic latency (may be years)
Stage 3	AIDS-related complex (ARC)
Final stage: AIDS	May have Kaposi's sarcoma (cancerous skin lesion) or *Pneumocystis jiroveci* (formerly *carinii*) infection (severe pneumonia); patient has no immunity

YOUR NOTES

_____

_____

_____

_____

_____

_____

_____

Specimen Collection and Handling

- Before collection:
  - Verify the identity of the patient (1st and last name, date of birth).
  - Review the requisition slip and confirm the patient's proper test preparation.
  - Assemble the needed collection equipment and supplies.
  - Wash hands before and after each procedure.
  - Wear gloves when appropriate.
  - Micropuncture and venipuncture sites are cleansed with alcohol. Use the spiral technique, working from inside to outer edges. Allow the site to air dry or dry with sterile gauze.
  - Use sterile collection containers and equipment.
- After collection:
  - Label the container with the patient's name, date, time of collection, specimen source, and your initials.
  - Use a biohazard-labeled bag or puncture-proof container to dispose of all hazardous waste.
  - Incubate culture plates with the agar side up, so moisture droplets will not fall on the growing surface.

- Handling
  - Store the specimen according to instructions: refrigerate, separate blood components, and so forth.
  - Avoid contaminating (soiled, stained; inferior or impure by admixture) specimen or oneself.
  - Transport disease-causing microorganisms using agar (sheep's blood) as a medium to ensure nutrition for microorganisms.

Urinalysis

A thorough routine urinalysis may provide more information about the general condition of the body than any other set of tests.

The kidney filters about 1,000 L of blood a day; the average adult produces 1,250 mL/day (1.25 L). Urine is composed of 95% water and 5% waste products. It is usually sterile, meaning it does not contain bacteria or other infection-causing organisms.

Collection

- The specimen must be tested as soon as possible.
  - If unrefrigerated, test the well-mixed specimen within 1 hour.
  - If refrigerated, wait until the specimen is at room temperature (no more than 2 hours).

Collection Techniques

- **Random**
  - Most common sample type
  - Used for routine screening
  - Collection of 3 oz or more
- **1st morning specimen**
  - Has the highest solute concentration; used in pregnancy testing for human chorionic gonadotropin (HCG)
  - Has the highest specific gravity

- **Fasting sample**
  - Second morning specimen
  - A must for diabetic monitoring
- **Clean-catch midstream**
  - Best for bacterial culture and culture and sensitivity (C&S) testing
  - Analyzes for type of bacteria and identifies best antibiotic to use
  - Inside of container kept sterile and as free as possible of bacteria surrounding the urethra
- **24-hour**
  - For quantitative analysis
  - Study of calcium, potassium, creatinine, urea nitrogen, protein, and lead levels
  - Collection begun after the 1st morning void
- **Catheterization**
  - Collected if the patient cannot urinate normally
  - Performed if the specimen must be completely sterile

Analysis

Physical Examination

- **Color:** Pale straw to dark amber
- Other color indicators:

Urinalysis	
Color	Possible Causes
Colorless	Drinking excessive amounts of water
Red	Blackberry, cranberry, beet consumption; blood (kidney or bladder infection, cancer, trauma)
Neon yellow	B-complex vitamin, excess riboflavin (B_2)

Continued

Urinalysis—cont'd	
Color	**Possible Causes**
Orange	Pyridium (drug to treat bladder infection)
Dark yellow	Dehydration; early sign of liver problem
Brown	Bean (especially fava) or rhubarb consumption; old, disintegrated blood clots
Blue	Methylene blue (drug ingredient for bladder spasm and discomfort)

- **Clarity:** Rate from transparent to turbid (degree of cloudiness)
- **Specific gravity:** A density measurement compared with distilled water
  - Normal range: 1.005 to 1.030
  - Measured by urinometer, refractometer, or on a reagent strip
- **Odor**
  - A fruity odor indicates diabetes.
  - A foul odor indicates infection.
  - An ammonia scent indicates a high concentration of bacteria from sitting at room temperature too long.

Chemical Examination

- **Reagent pads**
  - They are located on strips that are dipped into the urine specimen.
  - Pads react by changing color.
  - Measurements taken are timed.
  - Measures the following:
    - The pH (potential hydrogen) scale (the acidity and alkalinity of a solution): normal range, 4.5 to 8.0; pH of 7, neutral; pH above 7, basic (alkaline); and pH below 7, acidic
    - Other pads

Reagent Pad	Abnormal Result Indicates
Albumin (protein)	• UTI • Kidney disease • Vigorous exercise
Bilirubin (degenerated RBCs)	• Points to liver damage • Obstructive jaundice • Hepatitis
Blood	• Kidney damage • Urinary tract disease • Severe burns • Muscle injury • Menstrual period in women
Ketone bodies (acetone)	• Fatty diet • Severe diabetes mellitus • Starvation • Dehydration • Exposure to cold • Excessive exercise
Glucose	• Possible diabetes mellitus if above renal threshold
Nitrate	• Pathogen presence (UTI) Note: False-positive result for nitrates may occur if the specimen is left out for more than 2 hours; bacteria create nitrite in vivo
Urobilinogen (converted bilirubin)	• Points to heart disease • Liver disease • Hemolytic anemia

RBCs, red blood cells; UTI, urinary tract infection.

Microscopic Examination

Microscopic urinalysis is not CLIA waived; a medical assistant must have additional training and meet CLIA 1988 quality-assurance protocols for the laboratory.

• Findings should correlate with the physical and chemical analyses. For example, if the presence of RBCs on the reagent strip is identified, then RBCs would be seen microscopically, and the urine specimen color would have a pink or red hue.

- Procedure
  - After centrifuging, pour off supernatant.
  - Set up a wet mount to examine urine sediment.
  - Unstained sediments are best viewed using high (40×) power and low light.
- Common structures found in urine are as follows:
  - **Epithelial cells:** Come from the genitourinary tract
    - Renal tubular cells
      - Morphology: Round, large nucleus
      - A high number present indicates tubular damage or acute infection (e.g., glomerulonephritis)
    - Transitional cells
      - Morphology: Round to oval, may have a tail
      - A high number present indicates bladder disease or renal pelvis disease.
    - Squamous cells
      - Morphology: Large, flat, irregular cells
      - A high number present indicates vaginal contamination in women.
  - **RBCs:** Normal, 0 to 2 cells seen using a high-power field (HPF).
    - Morphology: May be round, colorless, from hemolysis
    - An increased number present may indicate bleeding somewhere along the urinary tract.
  - **WBCs:** Normal, 0 to 5 cells seen using an HPF.
    - An increased number present may indicate inflammation of the genitourinary tract.
  - **Crystals:** Common in all urine specimens; especially if allowed to cool
    - Type and number vary with the pH of the urine specimen.
    - They are not usually clinically significant unless found in large numbers (amorphous crystals).

- Abnormal urine crystals: Possible causes are disease states, inherited metabolic disorders, medication, or treatment.
  - Cystine (6-sided) indicates calculi or a congenital defect; it can cause mental retardation.
  - Uric acid indicates gout.
  - Tyrosine needle and leucine spheroid indicates severe liver disease.
  - Cholesterol indicates severe UTIs.
  - **Mucus threads:** Normally present in small amounts in the urine; long, wavy threads with pointed ends
  - **Spermatozoa:** Common in both men and women
- Uncommon structures found in urine are as follows:
  - **Bacteria:** Should not normally exist in the urinary tract. The presence of more than a few indicates specimen contamination or a UTI.
  - **Parasites:** *Trichomonas vaginalis* is a common parasite.
  - **Yeast:** This indicates a diabetic patient or vaginal contamination caused by *Candida albicans* (candidiasis).
  - **Casts:** These are cylindrical structures formed in the lumen of nephron tubules within the kidney.
    - Casts are made up of hardened materials within the lumen that are flushed out into the urine. Their presence generally indicates a diseased condition.
    - They are counted under a low-power field (10×) and low light and are identified under an HPF (40×).
    - The types of casts are named for their structural material.
      - **Hyaline casts:** Pale, colorless cylinders with rounded edges. They indicate kidney disease or are seen as normal in response to heavy exercise.
      - **Granular casts:** Either coarse or finely granular in appearance. They indicate heavy proteinuria, acute or chronic renal disease, or congestive heart failure (CHF).
      - **Cellular casts:** They are named for the organized structures they contain.

- **WBC casts** indicate pyelonephritis (chronic renal disease).
- **RBC casts** indicate pathological conditions: acute glomerulonephritis, lupus nephritis, and severe nephritis.
- **Renal tubular epithelial casts** indicate ischemia.
- **Waxy casts** indicate severe renal disease.

YOUR NOTES

_____

_____

_____

_____

_____

_____

_____

Hematology: Analysis of Blood

Blood is the transportation system in the body. Blood content is examined and tested to give general health information and to identify disease-causing organisms. Medical assistants may perform a blood cell morphology examination, cell counts, and various chemical analyses.

Three types of specimens can be obtained from a venous blood sample:

- **Serum:** Sample blood is collected in a tube without an additive. Once collected, the blood is left standing in an upright position at room temperature, usually for 10 to

30 minutes to allow a clot to form. Serum is the watery portion of the blood that contains the antibodies, and it does not contain any clotting factors. Serum is used most frequently for blood chemistry tests, pregnancy tests, viral studies, and the HIV antibody test.

- **Whole blood:** Sample blood is collected in a tube with an anticoagulant additive. It is used most frequently for hematology tests such as a complete blood count (CBC), coagulation studies, blood glucose, and some other blood chemistry tests.
- **Plasma:** Sample blood is obtained from whole blood collected in a tube with an anticoagulant additive and is then centrifuged. Plasma is 90% water and 10% proteins, carbohydrates, fats, amino acids, mineral salts, hormones, gases (carbon dioxide [CO_2] and O_2), antibodies, enzymes, and waste (urea, uric acid). Centrifugation causes the specimen to separate into 3 layers. The top layer is plasma, the middle layer contains WBCs and platelets ("the buffy layer"), and the bottom layer contains RBCs. Hematology tests and some chemistry tests are performed on this type of specimen.

Blood

- Whole blood's total volume is 55% plasma and 45% formed elements.
  - **Plasma**
    - 90% water; 9% protein; 1% fats, carbohydrates, gases, waste products, clotting factors, and minerals
  - **Formed elements**
    - RBCs (erythrocytes), WBCs (leukocytes), and platelets (thrombocytes)
    - Cells formed mostly in red bone marrow
    - **Reticulocytes:** Newly released RBCs from bone marrow; circulate in peripheral blood for 24 to 36 hours as reticulocytes before becoming mature RBCs; normally, make up 1% of peripheral RBCs

- **White blood cells:** There are 5 types of WBCs, which fight infections:
  - **Agranulocytes** (formed in lymphatic system)
    - Lymphocytes
    - Monocytes
  - **Granulocytes** (formed in red bone marrow)
    - Neutrophils (most numerous)
    - Basophils
    - Eosinophils

Leukocytes

Granulocytes	Nongranulocytes

Neutrophils
58%–66% of WBCs

- Fight bacterial infection by phagocytosis
- Primary defense against infection

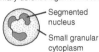

Segmented nucleus

Small granular cytoplasm

Lymphocytes
21%–30% of WBCs

- Produce antibodies to foreign antigens
- The "backbone" of the immune system

Large nucleus

Basophils
0%–1% of WBCs

- Fight allergies
- Use phagocytosis
- Secrete heparin, histamines, serotonin

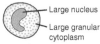

Large nucleus

Large granular cytoplasm

Monocytes
Largest WBC
4%–8% of WBCs

- Eliminate dead fragments, dead cells
- Use phagocytosis
- Produce interferon

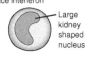

Large kidney shaped nucleus

Eosinophils
2%–4% of WBCs

- Fight allergies and parasitic infections
- Use phagocytosis

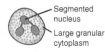

Segmented nucleus

Large granular cytoplasm

White blood cell types and functions.

Blood Collection Techniques

Micropuncture (Fingerstick)

- Follow the appropriate steps noted previously in "Before Collection" under "Specimen Collection and Handling" (page 323–324).
- Select the (great) middle or ring finger of the nondominant hand. On infants, use the underside of the outer edge of the heel.
- Cleanse with an alcohol pad; allow to dry or wipe with a sterile gauze pad.
- Puncture should be no deeper than 2.4 mm (0.1 inch).
- Wipe away the 1st droplet of blood because it contains more tissue fluid.

Venipuncture

- This is most commonly performed for hematological testing.

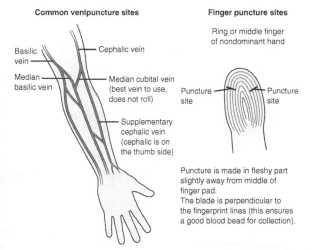

Common venipuncture sites

Basilic vein

Cephalic vein

Median basilic vein

Median cubital vein (best vein to use, does not roll)

Supplementary cephalic vein (cephalic is on the thumb side)

Finger puncture sites

Ring or middle finger of nondominant hand

Puncture site

Puncture site

Puncture is made in fleshy part slightly away from middle of finger pad.
The blade is perpendicular to the fingerprint lines (this ensures a good blood bead for collection).

Common venipuncture sites and finger puncture sites.

- The most common site is the median cubital vein; other commonly used sites are as follows:
  - Cephalic (thumb side on forearm)
  - Basilic veins and back-of-hand veins
- **Venipuncture sites to avoid**
  - Extensive scars from burns and surgery
  - Veins subject to numerous punctures
  - Upper extremity on the side of a previous mastectomy
  - Hematoma
  - Edematous extremities
  - IV therapy and/or blood transfusions
  - Arm with a fistula or cannula
- **Needles**
  - Usual gauges for venipuncture are 19 to 23.
  - The higher the gauge number, the higher the risk of hemolysis.
  - For the butterfly technique, a 21- to 25-gauge needle is used.
    - This technique is used for small veins and on geriatric, pediatric, and burned patients; patients with limited range of motion, and patients receiving frequent needlesticks.
- **Collection tubes**
  - Adults: Usually 3- to 10-mL tubes
  - Children: Usually 2- to 4-mL tubes
  - Tube color determined by tube content
- **Venipuncture steps**
  - Follow the appropriate steps noted previously in "Before Collection" under "Specimen Collection and Handling" (page 323–324).
  - Apply a tourniquet 3 to 4 inches above the planned puncture site, have patient make a fist, and palpate the site.
  - Release the tourniquet, cleanse with an alcohol pad, and allow to dry or wipe with a sterile gauze pad.
  - Reapply the tourniquet.
  - The tourniquet must be released within 1 minute.
  - Anchor the vein below the intended site.

- Enter the vein with the needle bevel up, at a 10° to 15° angle.
- Release the tourniquet when blood flow is established.
- Remember the correct "order of draw."
- Gently invert each specimen tube 5 to 10 times (tipping to 1 side counting as 1 count) to thoroughly mix the collected blood with any additive within the tube.

Recommended Order of Draw

Conventional Color Stopper	Glass Tube Contents	Tests or Studies
1st: Yellow or yellow/black	Sodium polyanethol-sulfonate (SPS)	Blood cultures in microbiology; blood bank studies
2nd: Red	None	Serum chemistry studies; immunology studies; blood clotting time; blood bank
3rd: Red/black (tiger)	Serum separator tube: serum gel separator, clot activator	Serum chemistry studies
4th: Light blue (not drawn 2nd if there is a concern regarding contamination by tissue fluids or thromboplastins)	Sodium citrate	Coagulation studies
5th: Green	Sodium heparin, lithium anticoagulant	Plasma chemistry studies; lithium or ammonia level; arterial blood gases

Continued

Recommended Order of Draw—cont'd		
Conventional Color Stopper	Glass Tube Contents	Tests or Studies
6th: Lavender, pink	EDTA, anticoagulant	Whole blood hematology (CBC, WBC); whole blood immunohematology testing; lead studies; sedimentation rate
7th: Pale yellow	Acid citrate dextrose A and B	HLA tissue typing; paternity testing; DNA studies
8th: Gray	Potassium oxalate or sodium fluoride (glycolytic inhibitors), anticoagulants	Glucose studies (GTT, FBS); lactic analysis; blood alcohol levels

CBC, complete blood count; EDTA, ethylenediamine tetra-acetic acid; FBS, fasting blood sugar; GTT, glucose tolerance test; HLA, human leukocyte antigen; WBC, white blood cell.

- **Difficult venipuncture**
  - **Failed attempts**
    - If the 1st attempt fails to collect the specimen, remove the needle, and try the other arm.
    - If the 2nd attempt fails, change the needle position, try using another tube, and loosen the tourniquet.
    - After the second attempt fails, call another experienced phlebotomist to help.
  - **Loss of blood flow into the tube**
    - This may be caused by vein collapse.
    - Resecure the tourniquet to increase filling.
    - Remove the needle to redraw.
    - Reposition the needle; it may no longer be in the vein.

- **Additional venipuncture information**
  - **Hemolysis:** The rupturing of RBCs causing the release of hemoglobin (Hb [also abbreviated Hgb]) into the blood specimen. In phlebotomy, causes may be as follows:
    - Needle gauge used is too small
    - Shaking the collection tubes
    - Drawing blood before alcohol is dry
  - **Hemostasis: The stoppage of bleeding in a damaged blood vessel**
  - **Flash:** The 1st appearance of blood drawn into a vacuum tube, tube, or syringe during the venipuncture procedure; gives confidence to the phlebotomist

Whole Blood Analysis

- **Blood counts:** These quantitative studies look at the total number of blood cells and the percentage of each type of cell that makes the entire sample.
  - CBC
  - RBC count
  - WBC count
  - WBC differential (percentage of each type of WBC)
  - Platelet count (automated)
- **Blood cell morphology:** This analyzes the shapes, sizes, and possible groupings of the cells.
  - The study is possible by creating a blood smear.
  - A blood smear is from a fresh blood specimen containing an anticoagulant and then prepared on a glass slide by applying a drop of blood to the slide. A spreader slide is used to pull the blood thinly on the slide. The slide is then stained to complete preparation and examined under a microscope. This process is also done to perform a WBC differential count.
- **Hemoglobin (Hb):** A quantitative analysis of the protein within RBCs containing iron. The iron attracts and binds O_2, which is then transported to body tissues.
  - Hb is the main component of an RBC.
  - Normal range in men is 14 to 18 g/dL; in women, it is 12 to 16 g/dL.

- **Hematocrit (Hct):** A measurement of the percentage by volume of RBCs in whole blood (after it has been centrifuged).
  - The normal range in men is 42% to 52%; in women, it is 37% to 47%.
  - Duplicate Hct results should not vary by more than 2% of each other.
  - Layers in centrifuged (spun) Hct are (from top to bottom) plasma, "buffy coat," and packed RBCs.
  - The ratio of Hct to Hb in people is generally 3:1. Multiply the Hb value by 3, and round this number to the nearest whole number; use the formula

  $$Hb \times 3 = Hct + \text{ or } - 3.$$

- **Bleeding time:** Evaluates the blood's ability to clot; the normal range is 2 to 7 minutes.
- **Blood typing and ABO antigens:** Agglutination points to the type of blood.

	Blood type	Antigens/ antibodies	May donate blood to	May receive blood from
A antibody, B antibody	O+	Rh+ is antigen D; anti-A and anti-B antibodies	O+, A, B, AB	O
	O− (rare)	No antigens No antibodies	Universal donor	O−
A antigen, B antibody	A (most common)	A antigen/ anti-B antibodies	A, AB	A, O
B antigen, A antibody	B	B antigen/ anti-A antibodies	B, AB	B, O
A antigen, B antigen	AB (rarest)	A and B antigens/ no antibodies	AB	Universal recipient

ABO blood grouping.

- **Rh factor:** D antigen found on the RBC surface
  - If an RBC contains the Rh factor, then it is Rh+; without the factor it is called Rh–.
  - If an Rh– person's blood is given to Rh+ blood, then it becomes sensitized and develops anti-Rh antibodies. If this same person is given Rh+ blood again, then the anti-Rh antibodies will attack (by agglutinating) the Rh+ blood.
  - About 85% of the population is Rh+.
  - **RhoGAM** is given to Rh– women who have just given birth to prevent the possible Rh+ blood of the newborn from triggering the development of anti-Rh antibodies. This is done to ensure that the 2nd baby and future babies will not develop **erythroblastosis fetalis.** This condition is life-threatening to the newborn.
- **Erythrocyte sedimentation rate (ESR or sed rate):** The rate at which RBCs settle to the bottom of a blood specimen. RBCs are the heaviest of all the blood's components.
  - It is measured in millimeters per hour (mm/hr).
  - It determines the degree of inflammation in the body.
  - The Wintrobe and Westergren methods are used.
- **Glucose:** Chemistry test; normal range, 70 to 110 mg/dL
  - Fasting blood glucose (FBG)
    - 12-hour fast, except water
    - Above normal test results, glucose tolerance test (GTT) needed
  - **GTT** (glucose tolerance test)
    - Timed
    - Routine at 6 months of pregnancy
  - **HbA1c**
    - Used to monitor patients with diabetes
    - Measures the amount of glycosylated Hb (glucose molecules attached to Hb) in the blood
    - Reveals diabetic patients' compliance with prescribed diabetes treatment
- **Carbohydrate metabolism**
  - In preparation, the patient eats a high-carbohydrate diet for 3 days and fasts 8 to 12 hours before the test. The patient may have a little water.

- The 1st blood draw should be less than 150 mg/dL, after which glucose is given orally.
- Half an hour later, blood and urine are drawn each hour as the MD prescribes.

- **Cholesterol**
  - Cholesterol—a white, waxy, fatlike substance (lipid)—is essential for normal function of the body.
  - It is an important component of cell membranes.
  - It is used in production of hormones and bile.
  - Normal total cholesterol should be less than 200 mg/dL.
  - Low-density lipoprotein (LDL) should be less than 130 mg/dL.
    - **LDL** is commonly called **bad cholesterol.**
    - It picks up and carries fats to the blood vessels and causes plaque to build up on the arterial walls, with resulting atherosclerosis.
  - High-density lipoprotein (HDL) should be greater than 35 mg/dL.
    - **HDL** is commonly called **good cholesterol.**
    - It removes excess cholesterol from the cells and carries it to the liver to be excreted.
  - **Triglycerides**—a blood fat related to the risk of heart disease—should be less than 250 mg/dL.

Guaiac (Occult) Blood

- This test is used to detect hidden bleeding in the gastrointestinal (GI) tract.
- A stool sample is collected by the patient and applied to a reagent paper.
- The health-care provider receives the sample and appropriate measures are taken if the test result is positive.

Test	Normal Values	Above Normal Results May Indicate	Below Normal Results May Indicate
Creatinine	4-1.5 mg/dL	• Impaired renal function • Chronic nephritis • Urinary tract obstruction	• Muscular dystrophy
Blood urea nitrogen (BUN)	8-25 mg/dL	• Kidney disease • Urinary tract obstruction • Borderline high • Congestive heart failure • Internal bleeding	• Liver failure • Negative nitrogen balance • Impaired absorption (celiac disease) • Overhydration • Low-protein diet
Uric acid	Male patients: 3.5-7.2 mg/dL Female patients: 2.6-6 mg/dL	• Gout • Chronic kidney failure • Kidney stones • Radiation poisoning • Toxemia of pregnancy • Starvation • Diet rich in purines (organ meats)	• Not significant

Continued

Test	Normal Values	Above Normal Results May Indicate	Below Normal Results May Indicate
Total protein	6–8 g/dL	(From dehydration from loss of body fluids) • Lupus erythematosus • Rheumatoid arthritis • Chronic infections • Acute liver disease	• Severe liver disease • Malabsorption • Nephrotic syndrome • Diarrhea • Exfoliative dermatitis • Severe burns
Total bilirubin	0.3–1.2 mg/dL	• Liver disease • Bile duct obstruction • Hypothyroidism • Borderline high • Jaundice	• Drug addiction (barbiturates)
Alkaline phosphatase	30–115 milliunits (mU)/mL	• Gallstones • Liver lesions • Hepatitis • Cirrhosis of the liver • Paget disease • Metastatic bone disease • Osteitis deformans	• Osteomalacia • Malnutrition • Hypothyroidism • Pernicious anemia • Scurvy • Placental insufficiency

Serum aspartate aminotransferase (AST)*	Children: 10–50 units (U)/L Infants: 20–60 U/L	• Myocardial infarction • Severe arrhythmias • Severe angina • Cirrhosis of the liver • Acute hepatitis • Infectious mononucleosis • Hepatic necrosis • Acute pancreatitis • Acute hemolytic anemia • Acute renal disease • Severe burns • Muscular dystrophy	• Beriberi • Uncontrolled diabetes mellitus with acidosis
Serum alanine aminotransferase (ALT)*	Adults: 7–56 U/L Children: 10–35 U/L	• Hepatocellular disease • Obstructive jaundice • Active cirrhosis • Metastatic liver tumor • Mild pancreatitis • Liver congestion • Hepatic injury in myocardial infarction	• Not significant

*If AST is high and ALT is normal, patient had a heart attack, not liver damage. If both AST and ALT are high, patient has liver disease.

Serology (Immunology)

Immunology is the study of the body's defenses against foreign substances. Serology is the scientific study of the fluid components of blood, especially the measurement of reactions between antigens and antibodies within blood serum. Antigens and antibody testing may also use urine and body fluids.

- Antigens are substances considered foreign by the body's immune system (e.g., a cancer antigen [a protein or carbohydrate released by cancer cells] or a disease-causing microorganism).
  - The presence of an antigen causes the immune system to create antibodies against it.
- Antibodies flow freely through blood and are found in blood serum.
- The presence of antibodies is measured by a **titer.**
  - Specifically, a titer measures the presence and concentration of a substance (e.g., hormones, vitamins, drugs). For example:
    - **Hormone detection** (e.g., pregnancy tests for HCG)
    - Titers also used in ABO and Rh blood typing
  - Titers assist in the diagnosis of bacterial and viral disease such as:
    - Duodenal ulcers: 90% *(Helicobacter pylori)*
    - Infectious mononucleosis (Epstein-Barr virus)
    - Lyme disease (infected tick)
    - Streptococcal throat *(Streptococcus pyogenes)*
    - Rheumatoid arthritis
    - HIV
    - Influenza virus

The Electrocardiogram and the Cardiac Cycle

The ECG is most frequently performed for the diagnosis of heart disease. The abbreviation ECG is preferred over EKG. The term EKG was coined by Willem Einthoven, a

Dutch physiologist, in the late 1800s, when he developed the techniques to record the heart's electrical activity.

It is the medical assistant's responsibility to perform this test accurately and skillfully to ensure a correct reading. The equipment must be set up properly, electrical interferences must be corrected, adjustments must be done, and the patient's comfort (physically and mentally) must be seen to before performing the ECG.

Brief Description of a Complete Cycle

* A complete cycle is 0.8 seconds.
* The cycle is regulated by electrical impulses transmitted through heart wall tissues.
* The 4 heart chambers contract **(depolarization)** and then relax **(repolarization)** at different times.
* The atria contract 1st, followed by the contraction of the ventricles.
* The contraction of the ventricles moves blood out of the heart and into the body.
* **Normal rate of rhythm** (RR) is 60 to 100 beats per minute.

Detailed Description of a Complete Cycle

* **Diastole** (rapid filling phase)
  * **1st phase**
    * Atria receive blood from the superior and inferior vena cava and coronary sinus.
    * Ventricles have expelled all their blood into the aorta.
    * Pressure causes the atrioventricular (AV) valves to open (tricuspid and mitral).
  * **2nd phase:** Pressure in the atria and ventricles begins to equalize.
  * **3rd phase**
    * Atria contract to push out the last remainder of blood.
* **Systole** (QRS wave)
  * **1st phase:** Ventricles are full and begin to squeeze down on themselves to build pressure inside to force the semilunar valves to open.

- **2nd phase:** The semilunar valves open.
- **3rd phase:** Ventricular contraction continues until the last of the blood exits.
- **4th phase:** The ventricles relax.

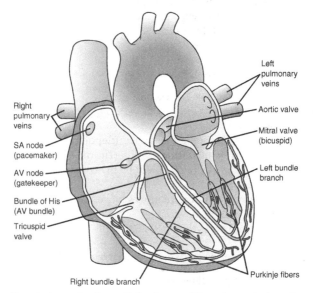

Electrical conduction of the heart. AV, atrioventricular; SA, sinoatrial.

- **Sinoatrial node (SA node;** the pacemaker)
  - The SA node generates the electrical impulse that activates the cardiac cycle.
  - It is responsible for atrial contraction.
  - It also triggers AV node action.
  - It controls the rate of heart contraction.
- **AV node** (the gatekeeper)
  - The AV node briefly delays the impulses from the SA node.
  - This delay keeps the ventricles from contracting too soon.

- The delay allows the atria to contract completely, to get all blood out and flowing into the ventricles.
- The AV node passes the impulse at 46 to 60 beats per minute.
- **Bundle of His**
  - The Bundle of His is triggered into action by the AV node.
  - It carries the impulse to the **left** and **right bundle branches** and eventually to the **Purkinje fibers.**
  - The bundle branches and Purkinje fibers are responsible for ventricle contraction.
  - The rate of ventricle cell contraction is 20 to 40 beats per minute.
- **Final phase**
  - The heart relaxes **(repolarization)** during the final stage.

ECG Monitoring

Holter Monitor

- This is used for patients experiencing intermittent chest pain or discomfort but who had normal results on a resting ECG.
- Depending on the need for and the type of Holter monitor, 3 to 5 leads are used to record cardiac activity over a 24-hour period or up to a few weeks to detect dysrhythmias.

The 12-lead ECG

- The 12-lead ECG uses 3 **bipolar** leads, 3 **unipolar** leads, and 6 chest leads **(precordial)** to record a heart's activity.
  - Bipolar leads (limb leads): The 1st leads read on an ECG
    - Lead I: Measures current traveling between the left arm and right arm = (LA-RA)
    - Lead II: Measures current traveling between the left leg and right arm = (LL-RA)
    - Lead III: Measures current traveling between the left leg and left arm = (LL-LA)

348 Part 3 Clinical

- Unipolar limb leads (AV means augmented voltage)
  - aVR: Right side; traces current traveling toward the right arm from midway between the left leg and left arm = RA − (LL + LA)
  - aVL: Left side; traces current traveling toward the left arm from midway between the right arm and left leg = LA − (RA + LL)
  - aVF: Foot; traces current traveling toward the left leg from midway between the right arm and left arm = LL − (RA + LA).

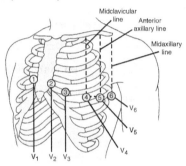

A 12-lead electrocardiogram on the upper chest.

Usual Lead Placement Sequence	Placement
V_1	At 4th intercostal space, right of sternum
V_2	At 4th intercostal space, left of sternum
V_4	At 5th intercostal space, midclavicular
V_3	At 5th intercostal space, midpoint between V_2 and V_4
V_6	At 5th intercostal space, left midaxillary line
V_5	At 5th intercostal space, midpoint between V_4 and V_6

- The right leg electrode is used as a ground electrode to minimize any possible electric shock to the patient and to stabilize the ECG. Traditionally, both the right and left leg electrodes are placed a few inches above the ankle on the fleshy part of the limbs. Alternate placement to reduce muscle artifact is on the upper leg as close to the torso as possible.
- The right and left arm electrodes are traditionally placed on any fleshy part of the arm. Alternate placement to reduce muscle artifact is midway between the elbow and the shoulder.
- Six chest electrodes are placed on the upper torso; 1 electrode is placed on each limb.

Heart Rate and Normal and Abnormal Rhythm

Most ECG machines display the patient's heart rate. Each P, QRS, and T-wave cycle represents a heartbeat, and time is measured on the horizontal axis.

Sinus rhythms originate in the SA node (the pacemaker). Sinus **bradycardia** occurs when the sinus rate is less than 60 beats per minute (common among athletes at rest). An exercising individual will exhibit a heart rate greater than 100 beats per minute, sinus **tachycardia**.

The terms **dysrhythmia** and **arrhythmia** are used interchangeably. **Dysrhythmia** is an abnormality in rhythm and **arrhythmia** is the absence of rhythm.

Rate, rhythm, and regularity are often considered together. A rhythm may be regular or irregular.

Common Sources of Error

- Poor skin preparation
- Loose connection to any electrode
- Patient's touching an electrode or any metal during recording

Artifacts

- **Somatic tremor:** Causes are body muscle movements such as coughing, sneezing, talking, or body shifting.

- **Electrical interference:** Causes are a poorly grounded machine, a machine placed too close to other electrical devices, or lead wires or cables that are exposed or broken.
- **Baseline interruption:** Causes are broken or dislodged leads.
- **Wandering baseline:** Causes are poor electrode skin connections movement of the cable and leads with respiration.

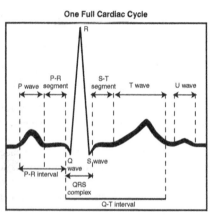

Reading the electrocardiogram.

The ECG Waves

- **P wave**
  - Represents depolarization of atria
  - Measures atrial activity
  - Seen as small, rounded, and upright
- **PR segment:** Part of atrial contraction
  - Between the P wave and the QRS complex
  - No electrical activity
- **P-R interval**
  - The time it takes the electrical impulse to be conducted through the atria and AV node to the beginning of ventricular contraction

- From the beginning of the P wave to the beginning of the QRS complex
- Measures the heart's efficiency at transmitting its impulses down the pathway
- **QRS complex**
  - Represents depolarization of ventricles
  - Atrial repolarization, usually not seen; occurs at the same time as the QRS complex
- **ST segment:** Part of ventricular contraction
  - Between the QRS complex and the T wave
  - No electrical activity
- **T wave**
  - Represents heart repolarization (relaxing)
  - Rounded, usually higher and broader than the P wave
- **U wave**
  - Late repolarization, not normally seen; should be shallow, rounded, upright

ECG Paper

- An ECG standardization mark is 10 mm high.
- If the baseline is off-center, the stylus position needs to be adjusted.
- ECG paper rolls out at 25 mm (1 inch) per second.
- The lines on the paper grid are 1 mm apart.
- Each small box represents 0.04 seconds.
- Each large box (5 small boxes across) represents 0.20 seconds.
- A cardiac cycle is represented by 4 large boxes (0.8 seconds).
- The RL (right leg) is not displayed because it is the ground electrode.

Pulmonary Function Tests

The pulmonary function tests (PFTs) measure the air taken into the lungs, the air expelled from the lungs, and how fast the air is pushed out of the lungs. The tests include spirometry, pulse oximetry, diffusion capacity, lung volumes, arterial blood gases, and cardiopulmonary exercise tests. They are used to assist in monitoring the effectiveness of treatments, and to classify and detect pulmonary problems such as chronic obstructive pulmonary disease (COPD), asthma, various allergies, chronic bronchitis, and cystic fibrosis.

- **Forced spirometry:** This simple, noninvasive screening test uses a spirometer to measure breathing capacity. It is the most frequently performed PFT.
  - **Forced vital capacity (FVC):** This maneuver measures lung capacity.
    - The patient inhales as deeply as possible and expels, in a rapid, forced expiration, the greatest possible volume of air into the spirometer.
    - The patient must continue to expel air for a total of 6 seconds.
    - The procedure must be repeated 3 times for accuracy in the evaluation.
    - The patient's sex, age, weight, and height are calculated factors affecting the normal expected test result.
    - A test result below 80% is abnormal.
  - Other lung capacity tests and definitions can be found in Chapter 3 in the discussion of the respiratory system (page 109).
  - Contraindications to testing include recent myocardial infarction (MI), angina, other serious medical conditions, smoking or eating a meal within 6 hours of test, viral infection or illness in past 2 weeks, and use of some medications that may affect test results.

Radiology

Radiology is the use of radiographic imaging to visualize and diagnose disease within the body. It is also the use of radioactive substances to treat diseases. In film radiography, an x-ray tube generates a beam of x-rays, which is aimed at the patient. The x-rays pass through the patient and strike undeveloped film, which is then developed and an image appears on the film. Radiography is often the 1st choice for imaging.

Common Radiographic Procedures

- **Computed tomography (CT)**
  - Produces a cross-sectional image of a body area; a series of x-rays is transferred to a computer, which puts together the cross-sectional view
  - Provides rapid, thin, detailed tissue planes
- **Intravenous pyelogram (IVP)**
  - Visualizes urinary structures and the colon
  - Uses iodine injection as the contrast medium
  - Patient preparation: Clear liquids the day before, then nothing by mouth (NPO) 8 hours before the test
- **KUB** (flat plate)
  - Frontal supine x-ray of the kidneys, ureters, and bladder
  - Used to diagnose abdominal complaints
- **Cholecystography**
  - Visualizes the gallbladder
  - Uses contrast medium
  - Patient preparation: No food or drink 12 to 14 hours before the test
- **Barium enema** (lower GI series)
  - Visualizes the lower portion of the GI system
  - Uses barium as the contrast medium
  - Preparation: Clear liquids the day before the test
- **Barium swallow** (upper GI series)
  - Visualizes the upper portion of GI system
  - Uses barium as the contrast medium
  - Patient preparation: NPO 8 hours before the test
- **Angiogram**
  - Visualizes the heart and circulation
  - Uses iodine dye, injected into a vessel using a catheter
  - Patient preparation: NPO 4 to 5 hours before the test
- **Arteriogram**
  - Visualizes the interior of arteries
  - Uses iodine dye, injected into an artery with a catheter
  - Patient preparation: NPO 4 to 5 hours before the test

- **Positron emission tomography (PET scan)**
  - Produces color images to assess metabolic or chemical activity
  - Uses radioisotope injection
- **Radiation therapy**
  - Treats disease (shrinks cancer tumors)

Other Imaging Methods

- **Magnetic resonance imaging (MRI)**
  - Produces views of internal structures (soft and hard tissues) without the use of radiation
  - No patient preparation needed
  - No metal objects worn or embedded (no mascara, no pacemaker)
- **Ultrasound (US)**
  - High-frequency sound waves producing images of deep body structures
  - Patient preparation, depending on the type of study:
    - No eating for several hours before the test (for pancreas, liver, gallbladder, and spleen examinations)
    - Drinking a specific amount of water and not voiding (for an obstetrical examination)
    - No eating for several hours before the examination and additionally taking a prescribed laxative and water with no voiding within an hour before the examination (for an abdominal examination)
  - US scan of the heart: **Echocardiogram**
  - The image produced by a computer: **Sonogram;** hard copy may be produced

Positioning for X-ray Pathways

AP (anteroposterior): Patient standing up or supine, beam guided from front to back

PA (posteroanterior): Patient standing up or prone, beam guided from back to front

RL (right lateral): Patient lying on right side, beam guided from left side to right side

LL (left lateral): Patient lying on left side, beam guided from right side to left side

Oblique: Patient lying at an angle, beam guided through body (left posterior or left anterior oblique, right posterior or right anterior oblique)

Safety and Protection for the Technologist, Assistant, and Patient

- **Monitored dosimeter:** A radiation exposure badge (a small device) worn by staff present during x-rays that monitors cumulative exposure to radiation. It is worn outside of clothing around the chest or torso. It monitors the dose received to unprotected parts (e.g., parts not covered with lead).
- **Lead shields:** These shields are used on patients to cover organs that do not need to be x-rayed (especially reproductive organs and the thyroid).
- **Pregnancy:** As a precautionary measure, female patients must be asked whether they could possibly be pregnant; if so, the radiologist must be notified before proceeding with the x-ray.
- **Equipment:** Maintenance of equipment should be scheduled regularly to ensure the equipment is in proper working order.
- **Lead aprons and gloves:** These are used by all participating staff members who are not behind a protective barrier during a procedure.
  - All participating staff should preferably be standing behind a barrier lined with lead when x-rays are being obtained.
- **Proper disposal:** All staff must follow the Occupational Safety and Health Administration (OSHA)–approved steps the facility uses to properly dispose of photo and x-ray processing waste, "hazardous waste," and "extremely hazardous" waste.

YOUR NOTES

_____

_____

_____

_____

_____

_____

_____

Sample Certification Test Questions

Now that you have studied this chapter, here are some sample certification test questions for you.

1. A patient suspects they are pregnant and has booked an appointment to come to the office. The medical assistant instructs the patient to bring in a urine specimen. Which type of specimen does the medical assistant tell the patient to collect?

   A. Random
   B. 24-hour
   C. First morning
   D. Clean-catch midstream
   E. Fasting

2. Immersion oil can be used with this microscope objective lens.

   A. 10×
   B. 100×
   C. 60×
   D. 200×
   E. 80×

3. What structure in the heart delays the electrical activity momentarily to allow the ventricles to complete filling?

  A. AV node
  B. Purkinje fibers
  C. SA node
  D. Bundle of His
  E. P wave

See the Appendix for the answers.

Remember to use Edge after you finish this chapter to test your knowledge. Directions for how to access Edge, as well as your access code, are located on the inside front cover of this text.

Answers to Sample Certification Test Questions

See the listed page for the answer's rationale.

Chapter 2: Medical Law and Ethics

1. **B:** page 47
2. **D:** page 38
3. **A:** page 40

Chapter 3: Anatomy, Physiology, and Medical Terminology

1. **D:** page 127
2. **C:** page 111
3. **E:** page 130

Chapter 4: Psychology and Interpersonal Communication

1. **B:** page 158
2. **A:** page 161
3. **B:** page 164

Chapter 5: Medical Office Administration

1. **B:** page 182
2. **A:** page 184
3. **D:** page 194

Chapter 6: Medical Insurance, Billing, and Coding

1. **D:** page 217
2. **C:** page 211
3. **B:** page 217

Chapter 7: Medical Office Communications

1. **C:** page 230
2. **D:** page 224
3. **E:** page 232

Chapter 8: Clinical Skills

1. **D:** page 257
2. **B:** page 247
3. **D:** page 261

Chapter 9: Pharmacology

1. **D:** page 293
2. **D:** pages 306 and 307
3. **B:** page 287

Chapter 10: Laboratory Diagnostics

1. **C:** page 224
2. **B:** page 316
3. **A:** page 346

Index

Note: Page numbers followed by "f" and "t" indicate figures and tables, respectively.